Praise for *Big Problems*

"Andy Boyle provides what's so often missing from health and diet advice: the sense that it's coming from a fellow human being who shares your plight. *Big Problems* is funny, earnest, and generous."

> —Dr. Ian Bogost, author, *Atlantic* contributor, and award-winning game designer

"A disarmingly breezy read. The hard science of weight loss—and gain—is interspersed with personal stories that will make you laugh out loud. It's the Cliff's Notes on exercise, food, and health you never knew you wanted."

> —Matt Wynn, investigative reporter for *USA Today*

"Andy Boyle strikes again! *Big Problems* is funny and accessible and ultimately inspiring."

> —Michael Kruse, senior staff writer for *Politico* and *Politico Magazine*

"Self-help books can be a drag—that's why Andy's book is so refreshing. The prose is crisp, fresh and funny, and devoid of pretension and judgment. The encouraging and funny tone is a welcome counterpoint to similar guides that may leave us feeling failure rather than realizing our own strengths."

> —John Wenz, science journalist and author of *The Lost Planets*

"What diet trend has piqued your curiosity? Workout fad? However you want to tame your waistline—fasting, CrossFit, fat freezing—Andy's tried it. This book opened my eyes to the cultural, scientific, and economic underpinnings behind why we eat the (generally crappy) way we do—and how all of us can pivot toward a healthier future."

> —Alex Richards, Pulitzer Prize finalist and assistant professor of journalism at Syracuse University

BIG
PROBLEMS

■ ■ ■

**A Former Fat Guy's Look at
Why We're Getting Fatter and
What You Can Do to Fix It**

■ ■ ■

ANDY BOYLE

A TarcherPerigee Book

**tarcher
perigee**

An imprint of Penguin Random House LLC
penguinrandomhouse.com

Most TarcherPerigee books are available at special quantity discounts for bulk purchase for sales promotions, premiums, fund-raising, and educational needs. Special books or book excerpts also can be created to fit specific needs. For details, write: SpecialMarkets@penguin randomhouse.com.

LIBRARY OF CONGRESS CATALOGING-IN-PUBLICATION DATA
Names: Boyle, Andy, author.
Title: Big problems : a former fat guy's look at why we're getting fatter and what you can do to fix it / Andy Boyle.
Description: New York : TarcherPerigee, [2020] | Includes bibliographical references. |
Identifiers: LCCN 2019044965 (print) | LCCN 2019044966 (ebook) |
ISBN 9780143133001 (trade paperback)
Subjects: LCSH: Weight loss—Popular works. | Food habits. | Health—Popular works. |
Nutrition—Popular works. | Physical fitness. | Exercise.
Classification: LCC RM222.2 (ebook) | LCC RM222.2 .B64829 2020 (print) |
DDC 613.2/5—dc23
LC record available at https://lccn.loc.gov/2019044965
p. cm.

Printed in the United States of America
1 3 5 7 9 10 8 6 4 2

To Maddie and Alex,
may you forever know you're loved

You are going to be short. You are going to be bald.
You don't have to be fat.

    —Dwight D. Eisenhower's dad (allegedly)

Eat food. Not too much. Mostly plants.

    —Michael Pollan

I'll eat that if you're done.

    —Me

Contents

Introduction

It was the middle of my first half marathon when I realized I was about to die.

People around me had started to drop like boulders amid the blistering Chicago summer heat. People who were in much better shape than me. People who actually looked like runners.

I had decided to run the Chicago Half Marathon—and do so much more—in order to learn extra about my body. In particular, I wanted to know how I had once gotten so fat. And why it was so hard to not be fat.

We should probably back up a little bit.

I used to be quite fat.

I mean, I still am, but I used to be, too. I'm just way less so now.

This is something I hear a lot from folks who weigh less than they used to: They always consider themselves overweight. These are people who run marathons, have washboard abs, and climb mountains for fun, and yet they still think of themselves as fat.

People who have achieved fitness feats most of us just dream about still look in a mirror and think something's wrong with them. Glad to know I'm in similar company with Olympians.

Years ago, I somehow managed to lose a lot of weight. (Depending on how you're counting, somewhere between eighty and one hundred pounds.) How I did it was nothing new: I watched what I ate. Exercise and my health became a regular part of my life.

I got rid of unhealthy habits, developed healthier ones, and changed my lifestyle around.

But at no point did I ever stop to wonder why: Why did I get so fat in the first place?

Why was I able to lose the weight—and keep the vast majority of it off—while many are not? Why is losing weight so hard? Why is fitness so hard?

Why is it so damn hard to get in shape?

This book is an attempt to look into the world of being, and trying not to be, overweight. Or, perhaps, what it means to be "in shape."

As a journalist, I have always strived to ask *why* about everything. And *how*. How come we, as a nation and a species, have gotten more overweight in the last hundred years? How come we're spending more money every year to combat obesity but not seeing any progress?

More than a third of Americans are considered obese. Another third are overweight. The statistics worldwide are about the same. It wasn't always like this, so what's different about now? Why is it so hard to get in better shape? What are we doing wrong when it comes to weight loss and health? What are we doing right?

I spent more than a year looking into these issues and writing about them. I experimented on my own body and tried different weight-loss plans, exercise routines, and diets. I met with doctors, weight lifters, and people of all shapes and sizes.

I discovered what it means to be in shape—from a scientific level as well as a personal one. Most important, I discovered, to some extent, why our brains are wired the way they are when it comes to fitness, food, and how we view our bodies.

You may be wondering, "Andy, what qualifies such a handsome person with an incredibly lush beard to write a book about fitness?"

Great question, and thank you for the compliment, dear reader. You're right: I'm no "qualified" expert. What I am is a former fat person who somehow managed to figure things out for myself.

I would include before and after photos of myself, but through the magic of your mind, just imagine the one on the left is a person who is much rounder than the guy you see in my author photo. Or to picture it more clearly, imagine me in a Coors Light shirt. I look kinda-almost pregnant, and my male-pattern baldness is quite apparent.

Guy on the right? Short buzz cut. Beefy arms. My belly is much smaller. I've got more of a V shape, and my striped shirt accentuates my skinniness.

This mental exercise proves I am good at both gaining *and* losing weight. That makes me *some* kind of expert. Or at least so I've decided. (I also learned that if you're balding, buzz your hair and/or wear hats.)

Most of the health and fitness books I see on the shelves are written by people who were always athletic, always made great food choices, and never seemed to struggle with their weight. They never experienced the frustration of being unable to find jeans at most stores. Or the sadness that comes when a stranger calls you fat on the street. Or the shame you feel after someone rolls their eyes or mumbles under their breath simply for the space your body takes up on a packed train or elevator.

Many of those authors never experienced not knowing where or how to start or the pain that comes with attempting something new that you feel utterly clueless at.

And then these people have the audacity to say, "I've never suffered like you, but just DO EXACTLY WHAT I SAY, AND IT'LL WORK FOR YOU."

Oh okay, dude.

I have felt the same pain the majority of overweight Americans have felt, mental and physical. I mean, I was the kind of fat where I regularly got told that I looked like every new famous fat, bearded person. That means I'm empathetic to their plight, and I want to help them in the same way I was able to help myself.

I hadn't ever seen a book written by someone who used to be huge—one that also deals with science, has funny personal anecdotes, and tries to keep a positive tone throughout—so I decided to write the book I wanted to exist when I was first figuring out my health and fitness.

On top of that, I'm a journalist. I've worked at newspapers and media outlets for more than a decade. My work has run in magazines. I even said "bare breast" on CNN Headline News one time. My mom was really proud of that.

I wanted to take that same journalistic lens and turn it inward. And then outward. And then inward again some more, just for good measure.

This book isn't a traditional *how-to* book when it comes to health and fitness. It's more of a *how-come,* with some helpful hints strewn about, especially at the end. I've peppered it with some stories in between all the science and research, just to keep things interesting.

I did all the extra sweating, injected myself with legal things (yup), attempted to freeze my fat off (also yup), and more so that perhaps you can learn a thing or two. I also made *a lot* of mistakes. (And managed to gain some weight back. And then lose it. And then gain it back. And then lose it. What fun!)

So yeah. I'm just a journalist on a journey toward becoming a better version of myself. And I want others to learn from my success, and from my failures, on my journey toward looking better in a T-shirt and learning to love my body.

Standard Warning

If you're suffering from any major medical ailments—mental, physical, anything—you should talk with a doctor before making any drastic changes to your lifestyle.

While I've tried to explain any inherent dangers in this book, know that changing your diet and adding exercise can be stressful on your body. Make sure your doctor gives you the go-ahead.

Another note: Unless your doctor has a practice that focuses on weight loss and fitness, maybe don't listen to their advice on how you should go about getting in shape.

1

Andy Got Fat

A STORY ABOUT MY UNDERWEAR

The most important day of my life involves my underwear.

The fateful day happened in the tail end of 2013. I was working for the *Chicago Tribune,* which is a thing called a newspaper. If you've never been inside a newsroom, let me describe it to you. Imagine an insurance office, except with shorter cubicle walls and sad people everywhere. Now imagine that everyone makes less money and is sadder.

There—you now know how every newsroom looks.

If you want to know your pecking order at a major American newspaper, the desk location they give you is a great indicator. If you're placed near windows with a view of the city, you're adored. If you're slammed into a windowless space with faulty air-conditioning, you're probably not well-liked. As for me, I was placed directly next to the men's restroom. Day in and day out, grumpy newspapermen would open the door three feet from me and do their business, with me basically guarding the door, like a member of the Night's Watch, except instead of defending the Wall, I was defending farts.

So now you know what my professional world was like.

Personally, I was in even worse shape. Literally. I was overweight, which is the nice way of saying I was fat. I know it may be hard to comprehend that, because you've looked at my author photo and you're thinking how gorgeous I am. For those of you trying to do the math and figure out whether I'm a 7 or an 8, I'm actually a 7.5. (Which, technically, rounds up to an 8.)

But back in 2013 I weighed 310 pounds, about 80 more than I do as of this writing. It was like I had a golden retriever shoved under my shirt. Except it couldn't play fetch, nobody wanted to pet it, and it was a bit hairier.

I was constantly sick. It seemed like every month I caught some new cold or developed bronchitis, and one time I had walking pneumonia, which led to a hazy trip to a nearby health clinic. I inquired why it was called walking pneumonia, and because our health care system in America is so great, the doctor shrugged, gave me a pamphlet, and told me to go to bed.

To recap: I was working in a depressing office. I was 300-plus pounds. I was sick all the time. And on this particular day, I was forced to sit in a meeting that was a waste of everyone's time. For those who have worked in an office, you know that a meeting is where productivity goes to die. And if you've read the Old Testament, you know that the first meeting of all time was in the Garden of Eden between Eve and the Serpent. So, meetings were literally created by the devil.

Whatever this meeting was about has been lost to the ages. But at some point during this work gathering, I crossed my legs underneath the conference room table. And somehow, because of the laws of physics and fabric, I did the most un-office-like thing ever.

I split my pants.

All I knew was I had moved my legs, and suddenly the world behind me had become quite drafty. I don't know if you've ever split your pants during a meeting at the *Chicago Tribune,* but it's hard to concentrate on anything afterward. All you're thinking is, "Oh crap, I split my pants, and I work at the *Chicago Tribune,* a place that gives me health insurance."

I reviewed my options. My first instinct was damage control. I couldn't let anyone know I ripped a hole in my britches. People at newspapers love to gossip. I would never be able to live that down. Knowing my odds, it would end up in the company-wide newsletter. Next, I had to figure out how to solve my pants problem. Perhaps I could run down the street to Target to pick up a new pair. (And if I did that, I'd end up buying twenty-seven more things.)

But I would need an excuse for why I had to leave work to shop at a store that's the height of Midwestern luxury. I imagined how that exchange would go with my manager.

"Boss, I gotta head out for a minute," I would say.

"How come?" he would ask.

"I split my pants, and my underwear is showing."

If you heard that, would *you* give me a raise?

At the end of the meeting, everyone got up to leave. And I stayed in my seat. The conference room was tiny, and the table in the middle took up 90 percent of the space. People were forced to awkwardly walk behind me, scrunched between my chair and the wall. Their faces showed their displeasure.

As he was leaving the cramped room, my boss finally said, "You, uh, okay, dude?"

He was a cool boss and called me "dude" sometimes.

And I answered, much too fast, "Oh yes I am fine, I just need to make a phone call, just a quick phone call, gotta go make a phone call, everything is fine, phone call, gotta make one."

My boss responded, "Uh, sure, dude." And he left. See? There's that "dude" again. Real cool guy, that boss.

I was now alone to contemplate my place in the universe, or at the very least, whether I would go through the rest of the day with my undies showing. It was time for me to strategize. I didn't know what to do, so looking to the wisdom of crowds, or at least a crowd of one, I texted a good friend of mine. It went like this:

"Ryan, let's say you have a friend, and your friend splits his pants at work. What should your friend do?"

Moments later, he texted back: "Is this friend yoooouuuuu?"

I texted him the sunglasses-wearing emoji for plausible deniability. Then I texted, "This isn't a time for jokes, Ryan. This is a time for answers and action."

He responded with a sentence that would change my life, a piece of advice that has stuck with me, and is at the same time the worst and the best advice I have ever received. He texted: "'Your Friend' should go across the street and buy some duct tape at Walgreens."

This is where our story takes a new turn. Because that's exactly what I decided to do. I managed to sneak out of the conference room and head straight toward the elevator, which was about thirty feet away. En route, I had to walk past the dozens of golden plaques for the Pulitzer Prizes the *Tribune* has won over the years. These awards are arguably the highest you can win in journalism. It felt like the eyes of history were upon my britches as I walked past them.

As I waited for the elevator, with my back to the wall, I saw four people approach me. Two of them were gigantic and in suits, wearing earpieces, obviously some sort of security. The third I knew worked for the newspaper's opinion section. You could tell because he was white and old.

The fourth person was also in a suit, was also white and old, and had this extra-pointless air about him, so I assumed he was a politician. He probably came to talk to the newspaper about important things, like a new tax cut for his rich friends, or yet another way to be sneakily racist.

But here I was, standing with my back facing the elevator doors, with a huge tear in my pants, like I was guarding the entrance. They all stared at me. Nobody said anything. All I could do was smile and pretend this wasn't happening.

When the elevator came, I quickly waddled in—backward, of

course. And during my backpedaling I *definitely* made eye contact with everyone. The security entourage gave me a quizzical look, and knew I wasn't going to be a threat unless there were cookies to steal. The politician didn't notice, probably because he was too busy thinking about what was best for women's bodies.

Eventually, we made it to the bottom floor, and I followed behind them, still trying to walk in a way that kept my bottom toward a wall at all times, lest anyone see my posterior shame.

Outside the building, I had to cross Michigan Avenue, one of the busiest streets in America. Hundreds of people were walking past, most with their phones out, ready to make a viral video. I leaned against the facade of the Tribune Tower, waited for the light to change in my favor, then sprinted across the street toward the Walgreens.

When I was just steps in front of the door, I tripped, falling in front of a gaggle of tourists who were watching a magician do close-up magic. I could only imagine what they saw: me, a giant man in a loud plaid shirt, facedown on the ground, my pants featuring a foot-long rip on the backside, my Fruit of the Loom undies flapping in the wind, as the nearby illusionist asked, "Is this your card?"

And then the card would appear stitched into the left cheek of my underwear, and people would lose their freaking minds.

Anywho, back in reality, I contemplated staying on the ground and never getting up. What if I lived in front of the Walgreens now? This could make a suitable home. Me and the magician could become close friends and go on adventures together. Instead, I gathered myself up and sauntered inside.

I was deeply exasperated and out of breath following my jog of maybe thirty feet. A cashier gave me an awkward glance, and then I asked simply, "Duct tape?" She pointed toward the back, I did the weird sideways walk, keeping my exterior pointed always toward a wall, away from anyone's eyeballs. I found the duct tape, purchased it, and did the same sprint back toward the Tribune Tower. Thankfully, this time, I did not fall.

I took the stairs up to the newsroom, knowing it would give me little chance of standing in an elevator with a famous person, having to explain why they could see my drawers. I exited and walked toward a less frequented men's restroom, a second one away from my desk. I hoped hitting up the least busy bathroom would mean I wouldn't run into anyone.

I was wrong.

As if fate were smiling upon me, an older reporter walked toward the bathroom at the same time as I did. As I was standing outside the door, trying to plan my escape from the man, he glanced at me. Then he looked at the duct tape in my hand.

He cocked his head and asked, "What are you doing going into the bathroom with duct tape?"

One of the most valuable lessons I've learned in life is that if you don't want to continue having a conversation, there's one phrase that always works, which is exactly what I said. I stared the man in the eyes and said, with utmost seriousness, "There's a situation."

And then, to give it added effect, I shook the duct tape in his general direction, like it was an emergency tambourine.

The reporter put his hands up and slowly sauntered away, not taking his eyes off me, realizing I must be, in fact, dealing with a situation. I snuck into the bathroom and found a stall. I immediately began fixing my situation.

You know that sound duct tape makes? That unmistakable duct tape sound? There's no other sound it could possibly be? Well, I was ripping off pieces of duct tape in this large bathroom when I heard a voice in the stall next to mine.

It boomed: "Is that . . . duct tape?"

I froze. I stopped breathing. I didn't want to answer, because then this person would hear my voice, be able to identify me in a voice lineup, and I'd have to explain to someone important why I had duct tape in the men's bathroom of the eighth-largest newspaper in America.

Eventually, the man washed his hands and left. I fixed my pants, duct-taping them on the inside, because while I may have been a slob, I at least knew to put the duct tape where people couldn't see it. My mom raised me well.

As I checked myself out in the mirror, examining the work I had done, a thought hit me hard. I hadn't looked at myself in a mirror like that in a long time, examining my entire body. I had gotten huge. Years of bad food, no exercise, and a lack of upkeep had taken their toll. And now I didn't like who I saw in the mirror. I barely recognized what I had become: an ever-fattening meat sack.

I knew I had to do something about the man I no longer recognized staring back at me. What I didn't know was how I would do it, but at least I had finally decided: This has got to stop.

I vowed I would never need to fix my pants with duct tape again.

Fun fact: Dear reader, I haven't used duct tape to fix an article of clothing since. I did use duct tape to fix a cat toy, which led to my cat getting duct tape stuck to him. Technically, that would make him a duct cat. Try saying that five times fast.

HOW DID I GET SO FAT? (AND THEN HOW DID I SLIM DOWN?)

Growing up, I heard the same thing from people about my weight: You're so smart! Why did you *let* yourself get so fat?

These were people who *loved me*, who felt the need to inform me that I was:

1. Fat
2. smart; but
3. still stupid because I got fat.

Super helpful.

Let's walk through a brief history of my life.

I was born in Sioux City, Iowa, because my hometown in Nebraska didn't have a hospital. (Still doesn't!) Thanks, Mom and Dad, for making me officially an Iowan until the day I die.

The small town I grew up in wasn't made for walking. If you wanted to go anywhere or do anything, you drove. (When I got older and could ride a bike, I did that whenever I couldn't trick my parents or older sister into driving me places.)

For breakfast, I had cereal—usually something sugary, Honeycomb being a particular favorite—and toast. For lunch, I ate whatever the school gave me (more on that later). For dinner, I usually ate with my family, but because both my parents worked, that occasionally meant fast food.

(This is not me blaming you, dear Mom and Dad; this is just me stating a fact. See, I am trying to show that this behavior is normal. It's all about setting a scene and making me relatable, Mom! Let me spin a narrative adventure here, okay?)

Exercise came in the form of running around the neighborhood, until my mom got AOL on our computer. Then all normal young-kid exercise stopped, and I sat on the internet from age ten until forever. Later, I would play sports but half-heartedly. I wanted to be on the internet, or reading a book, or doing something that didn't involve other human beings.

I was an artsy kid: band, choir, theater. On the side, I played in a bunch of *terrible* punk and/or ska and/or metal bands. I drove everywhere.

College happened, which mostly meant beer and excessive dining-hall food. Still, barely any exercise.

Graduation happened. A low-paying newspaper reporter job happened. More drinking because I was paid poorly and I had to live in Florida happened.

By the time I ended up in Chicago, in my late twenties, I was more than three hundred pounds. Most meals were fast food. Most liquids were soda. I walked more because I no longer had a car, sure, but I was still a hefty chunk of man meat.

Everything I've told you is the standard story of the modern human. Let's break it down.

Youth: They start with breakfast cereal, getting you addicted to sugar at a young age. After being pumped with commercials while watching cartoons, I craved whatever was the coolest new carbohydrate-enriched breakfast treat.

School: For, like, three straight years, my school lunch was from the "candy corner," which is where you could eat if you didn't want the "hot meal." I got a 3 Musketeers along with some nacho cheese and chips.

In high school, my lunch was usually some mass-manufactured burger or a slice of pizza. Sometimes milk.

In college, it was all-you-can-eat buffet style.

Exercise: Not much. I drove everywhere. I quit sports as soon as I got to high school. As I got older, I'd make plans in my head to exercise, but I was "too busy," which is millennial slang for "stayed at home and watched Netflix instead."

Alcohol: Oh yeah, I drank. Tons of calories. Then I'd get the alco-hungries afterward. (You're a smart reader, and therefore I'm going to let you figure out that portmanteau yourself.)

I knew *everything I was doing was bad for me.* I'm sure you feel the same way whenever you buy some candy or decide to eat something that's so processed it can't even be called "food"; they've got to give it some name like "milk treat" instead of "ice cream."

This is normal.

This is what has happened in our food system. It's become the fat-industrial complex. Almost everything in our country exists *to make you fatter.*

And because I live in this complex, I fell victim to it, just like millions (actually, *billions*) of other people. Maybe just like you!

I was able to turn it around. It wasn't easy. It still isn't easy. But I don't think the story of how I got so large is any different from most people's.

HOW I GOT LESS FAT

My story isn't unique. I was surrounded by unhealthy food, never developed healthy habits, and didn't know how to get out of the cycle of eat more, get fatter, feel sad, eat more, get fatter, feel sad . . .

Until one day, I did.

I think it all started when I decided to take a month off from drinking. The month prior I had the underwear incident you read about. I had also stepped on a scale, and the number was alarming.

I told myself, "I'm going to make two small changes: no drinking and only vegetarian food for a month." Now, to you, those may seem like gigantic changes. But in my head, I was like, "Okay, we're switching one thing off (alcohol), and moving other parts around (vegetarianism)."

After two days of being a vegetarian, I was starving. Then I googled "vegetarian hard what else," and pescetarianism popped up. Basically, a vegetarian who also eats fish. Seemed easier to follow.

That first month I had the best sleep and the most productivity— and I just felt better about myself. My self-esteem was up. My mood had improved. I didn't feel as regularly bitter as I *wanted* to be about everything.

At the end of the month, instead of going out for a steak and some Scotch, I decided to test myself: How long can I keep these healthy habits up?

A few months later, my clothes were fitting better. I stepped on a scale and was amazed I had lost weight. Next came more changes.

No more diet soda. I had long before stopped drinking regular pop—at least then I knew the disastrous effects of each can's monstrous amount of sugar. I took it out of my diet completely and switched to water and coffee.

I walked more. I had always enjoyed walking around wherever I lived, but now I set a goal. I'd try for a mile during my lunch break. I'd try for two miles after work. On the weekend, I would go for a two-hour urban hike in a new neighborhood.

Next, I cut out fast food for breakfast. (I know, shocking that this all worked, right?) Then I did some research and found healthier options for lunch near my office. For dinner, I found some easy meals I could make myself.

Did I always make my own breakfast and dinner? I did not. But was I more aware of the consequences of my food intake? You betcha.

But one huge thing happened more than anything else.

I liked myself again.

This may seem like a weird concept, especially for those who haven't dealt with their weight all their lives. The constant shame of being in a larger body can be debilitating. (See the chapter 8 section on weight bias.)

I often told myself, "What's the point of making any positive changes? You're always going to be fat. No one is going to like you. Why even try?"

Once I started to actually like myself—and like who I saw in the mirror—it became a lot easier to make more positive lifestyle changes, to modify my behavior in a way that led to more success.

That's got to start with you. Nobody can make you like yourself.

This is, of course, the easy answer of how I got fat and then less so. The harder answer? Well, we should probably start with a bit of history about being fat.

SELF-PRESERVATION AND MOTIVATION

My whole life is now a series of scheduled events meant to trick me into being less fat. If my brain had its way, I would sit on my couch, eat pizza topped with Cheez-Its and Cool Ranch Doritos, and never move.

2

How America—and the World—Got Fat

FAT USED TO BE COOL

For about four hundred years, until around 1900, being fat was pretty rad.[1]

The more you weighed, the more girth you had, the higher your status and the more beautiful you were perceived to be. Just look at all those paintings from that time period.

Are the most beautiful women of the ages depicted as being rail thin? Nope! Those gals got curves. Same goes for the powerful men of the era—the bigger the better.

Some of this change had to do with changing values in the predominant religion of the time, Christianity. (Maybe you've heard of it?) During the Middle Ages, the church was preaching how unimportant the flesh was. The less you had, the better you were. It meant you were living a pious life.

But during the Renaissance, things changed.[2] Being thin meant you were broke or sick. It also meant you weren't a partier, so to speak. This was a period of mental enlightenment as well as physical.

To be larger meant you were more down with whatever, in the parlance of our times.

Even in one medical textbook, it was said that carrying twenty to fifty pounds of "excess" flesh was healthy and a key part of vitality through any extended illness.[3]

This started to change during the early 1900s. The reasons are varied, but one was that insurance companies started to notice that obesity was linked with an earlier death. Then in the 1930s, the medical community started to change its tune: Excess fat was considered a health problem.

Fatness had also become associated with laziness. People started to act disgusted toward those who were perceived as obese, because it was viewed (and still is by many people) as some sort of moral failure.

For men and women, another thing happened: Corsets were going out of style.[4] This meant people's true sizes became known, and people were becoming more aware of their bodies.

Add to that the changes in media—film and television, as well as color photos in newspapers and magazines—which could quickly show idealized versions of the "perfect" male and female body.

And now we're where we are currently: Thinner is better, so the saying goes.

TECHNOLOGY AND THE CHANGING TIMES

If you want one big thing that's pushed us to be fatter, it's technology. Or rather, the way technology has changed our behaviors in the past hundred years.

Go outside for a minute. If you live in the country, this may be hard to do, but if you live in any sort of city environment, just go outside to the street. Turn your head left and then right.

How many cars did you see?

Probably a handful. And odds are, a few automobiles drove past you.

People walk a lot less than they used to. Some of this is because of the increase in suburbs and decrease in people living in larger cities, where you can use public transportation and walk to work or school or for fun.

But some of this is also because of the lack of easy access to places. Where I grew up in northeastern Nebraska, you more or less had to take a car to get anywhere. Sure, I could ride my bike to some places, but there wasn't any convenient public transit. My default mind-set was to hop in a car instead of walk.

Now that I live in the greatest city in the world (Chicago), I walk almost everywhere. I haven't owned a car in seven years. Do I take public transit? Sometimes. Do I rely a bit too much on ride-sharing apps? I do.

But I definitely walk a lot more than friends who've moved to the suburbs.

Our jobs

In 1970, almost a third of America's jobs were blue-collar, where people worked in manufacturing, mining, or construction.[5] Jobs where you were on your feet a lot, moved regularly, and had to use your arms and legs to get work done.

These kinds of jobs meant that people were burning a lot more calories throughout their day. Their daily caloric expenditure was much more than, say, someone who sits at his computer all day writing books about health and fitness.

But by 2016, the number of people who worked blue-collar jobs dropped to 13.6 percent of total employees. A lot of this is because of a drop in U.S. manufacturing jobs—many of those jobs have gone overseas, to countries where labor is cheaper and companies can make more money.

The number of people working in farming has also substantially declined. While agriculture never made up a giant portion of the

American workforce, in 1950 almost 10 million people were family farmers or hired help.[6]

In 2000, those numbers fell to almost 2.2 million. In part, new technologies have resulted in fewer people being needed to farm larger amounts of land. And also, advances in produce and livestock have meant that we have larger yields than we used to.

White-collar jobs have grown steadily, too. During the twentieth century, this type of labor went from 18 to 60 percent of the American workforce. Most of these jobs are in the service industry, and many are in offices.[7]

This means our workforce went from moving regularly to make stuff to sitting regularly to click and type stuff. And that means we expend fewer calories just to do our work as a nation.

I'm not here to discuss the merits of globalization and trade, but I am telling you this to point out one big thing: It means that we, as a country, move a lot less than we used to.

Exercise and movement burn calories. We have fewer jobs that require us to exercise and move. Just another factor that's led to all of us being bigger.

GREATER EASE IN BEING LAZY

Take the phone out of your pocket. No, actually do it. (Hopefully this book is still relevant in ten years, when phones are *implanted in our skulls* and we all walk around as iHeads.)

How many apps do you have that allow you to order food? I'm going to answer this right now with my phone. As a person who's always struggling with his weight, I currently have:

- Jimmy John's
- DoorDash

- Amazon (it can send food!)
- Instacart

Four. That's not too bad. OH, BUT WAIT—I also have Safari, my web browser. Can I log onto Grubhub? Yes. How about Domino's? Of course. Can I use my phone to call places and still get delivery that way?

You're damn right I can. Calling for delivery is an American right.

These sorts of apps are becoming ubiquitous, a regular part of our lives. And they're all mostly engineered to make you order more food.

With most food delivery services, you have some sort of minimum amount of food you need to order before you'll get a delivery. And because places are crafty, they'll make sure their prices don't make it easy to hit their minimum.

Case in point: A nearby restaurant I love but am sometimes too lazy to walk to has the best chicken burrito in America. (Fight me.) But all of their basic entrées are like eighty-nine cents below what you need for a delivery.

Do they have any eighty-nine-cent items? No—the next best thing is a two-dollar soda. But they also have chips and guacamole. Do I just get a two-dollar soda and call it good?

Of course not. I order the chips and guac, eat more than I ever wanted, and feel terrible the next day.

Ever try to order food online? You know what usually happens when you get to the end and you're about to check out: A pop-up asks if you'd like to add something else at a discounted price.

It's just like when you're at a fast-food joint and they ask if you'd like to make your meal a large, or add a crispy waffle or whatever new treat they're pushing on you. It *seems* like a deal because it's on sale. Our brains go, "Oh snap—I'm saving money." When in actuality, you're spending more money and consuming more calories.

DESIGN

It goes even further. Do you ever wonder why so many restaurant logos are red or orange? It's almost as if they all got together, had a vote, and were like, "Okay, nobody gets to use the blue!"

That's because research has shown that certain colors can make you hungrier, while others can suppress your appetite.[8]

It all goes back to evolution. Your brain registers certain colors as warning signs—black, purple, blue—for food that may be poisonous or rotten.

Guess what colors your brain thinks are inviting? Warm ones, such as red and yellow. (And a lot of these colors work *especially* well on kids, getting them hooked on processed food early in life.)[9]

And the next time you look at the colors restaurant owners use in their logos, advertising, and interior design, you'll see a trend: those same warm ones. It's not an accident.

It's almost as if they're using science to make you hungrier, eat more, and addicted to their food! *It's almost as if they're doing this.* (They're doing this.)

This is one reason blue plates are a good option if you're trying to limit your food intake. Although, there is some research that theorizes it's the contrast between the plate and food that helps you eat less, so the color blue may not be special, and the size of the plate and its color may have an impact, too.[10] Regardless, colors play an important shape in pushing us toward our food decisions.

ECONOMIC ISSUES

On top of how much technology has changed us, where we get our food has changed, too. Not everyone has easy access to fresh fruits and vegetables. In many parts of the United States, for instance, there are places called "food deserts"—communities that don't have a large grocery store or supermarket.

At least twenty-two communities qualify as food deserts in Chicago alone.[11] If you can't easily get healthy food, what are your options? Fast food. Food from corner stores. Lots and lots of processed, unhealthy things.

That kind of food, on the whole, is cheaper now than it used to be, partially because of advances in science and technology. And partially because the U.S. government spends billions to subsidize the additives that make this food cheaper, as well as billions to subsidize corn and soybeans, also regular ingredients used to make heavily processed foods.[12]

Healthy food, however? It's more expensive and also harder to find. But if you don't have access to it, how can you eat it?

And guess what parts of cities are most likely to be food deserts? Poor neighborhoods.

According to one study, counties in the United States with poverty rates higher than 35 percent have obesity rates that are 145 percent greater than those in wealthy counties.[13]

America's got a lot of poor people. As many studies have shown, people who start poor often stay poor. Which means they often stay in the communities they're from.

All this adds up to more reasons why more people are overweight in America. If we want to help fix the problem, we have to start fixing the problem of poverty, which, some would argue, is becoming even more exacerbated by technology.

This isn't an exhaustive list of how technology has changed us. It's just meant to give you more of the *how comes* and *whys* of the obesity epidemic in our country and our world.

I'm not some Ted Kaczynski–esque person who eschews all technology. Far from it: I've been writing code since middle school. I am using a computer to write this.

We have a society that's more technologically advanced now than at any time ever, and that progress is only going to continue.

We just need to stop and think what it's done to us, how all this has changed us, and how we haven't yet adapted to it. Not only that, but we need to realize how people are using technology against us—to make us heavier consumers, which in turn makes us heavier people.

NEW ORLEANS IS A BAD PLACE FOR A WEIGHT-LOSS CONFERENCE

During the hottest month of the summer, I decided it made sense to head down to New Orleans to learn more about obesity. No, this wasn't a trip to see how much shrimp I could eat (all of it), or how many beignets I could fit in my mouth at once (also all of them). It was to attend a conference about obesity.

I had never been to New Orleans before, nor had I ever attended a conference geared toward health issues. It was going to be an interesting event—one I hoped would open my mind.

It was run by the Obesity Action Coalition, or OAC, a nonprofit that was founded in 2005. Its story starts like this: A group of legislators got together and one asked who represented constituents affected by obesity. One realized there was a need for an organization like this to give these people a voice, and it was founded.

OAC currently has more than sixty-three thousand members and promotes creating a society that respects people who suffer from obesity, understanding the complex science around its causes and treatments, and giving help and guidance to those who are affected by the disease.

It's important you understand why I use that word—"disease"—to describe obesity. The conference talked about that a lot, and it changed my thinking on the subject.

Society tends to view obesity as this self-inflicted problem. You got fat because you made poor choices.

And, correlated with that, people usually make a *moral* choice about those who got fat, too. *You're a bad person because you are fat. You should know better.*

That's all a bunch of nonsense. Obesity is a chronic problem affecting millions of people for many reasons that are out of their control. (And if you believe otherwise, well, I hope you'll have changed your mind by the end of this book.)

OAC advocates for those affected by the disease, especially in the areas of discrimination, which happens in a lot of places, including in the workplace, schools, and doctors' offices.

OAC believes this, and I believe this, too: Nobody should be discriminated against because of their size or weight. Furthermore, people should have legal protections against these forms of discrimination.

Okay, now that that's out of the way, let me tell you a few of the more interesting things I learned.

Obesity affects people differently. On paper, I have been considered obese since I started college. I think many people who saw me wouldn't think that. (I have managed to get myself to the low end of merely "overweight" by medical standards through an extremely limited diet and heavy exercise, but still. I stayed at that weight for only a few months before I gained enough to put me back into obesity range.)

But when I attended the conference, I saw folks who were affected far more than me. Some folks had had bariatric surgery to actually decrease the size of their stomachs so that they would consume less food, which comes with a whole slew of other issues. Some folks had trouble moving because of their size, so they used wheelchairs and walkers to get around. And others, because of complications from obesity-related diabetes, were missing some of their extremities.

If anything, it made me aware of how lucky I was that I hadn't been affected as much as others. Or perhaps, because of my gender and my race, I had been given better treatment by doctors, or treated better by the world at large (we'll get to that), which helped me in the long run.

Pet obesity is also a problem. A lot of people who suffer from obesity also have obese pets. I'm no exception. My super fluffy cat, Tiberius, is a lot of fluff but also a bit of a mega-chonker. He's eighteen pounds, which, last time I talked with my vet, was about a 3.5 out of 5 in terms of health.

He's above where he needs to be. I've tried making him exercise more by playing with him, giving him diet food that requires a prescription (who knew you needed prescriptions for food?), and buying him food containers that required him to "hunt" for his food.

None of it worked. He's still a bit bigger. But the good news is, he's more or less been this size for years.

Is that bad? It depends. He's still active, he can still do what he needs to do, and, otherwise medically, he's still healthy overall. He's just bigger than doctors think he should be.

Sound familiar?

It helps to plot your weight gain on a timeline. One psychologist had everyone in the giant meeting hall take out a sheet of paper and write down what we remembered as our weight over time. When did we gain weight? When did we lose weight? Maybe we couldn't use exact numbers, but we could try to get a general sense of when things occurred.

Then she told us to think about what was happening in our lives. Bullied in school? Go through a messy breakup? A giant work project?

She had us point out when these stressful events occurred and then think whether our weight was affected by them. I stared at my graph—it was so clear. Every time I had ever managed to lose weight, it came back as soon as some new tragedy struck my life.

It was like you could just see it in action. Bullied throughout school. Weight gain. Stressful job after graduation. Weight gain. I manage to get a handle on things, make some better choices. Weight drops a bit. Death of my grandma. Weight gain.

It made me truly realize how much our stress and our mental health play a role in our weight, too.

All "fad" diets work. If you follow them, that is. One scientist showed us the results of multiple studies over many years. If you follow any of the leading "book" diets over time, these diets work.

Why? Because they usually trick people into eating fewer calories. Not only that, but they're getting more of their calories from protein and fats versus carbohydrates.

That's one reason the low-carb diets work so well—fewer carbs in general means fewer calories in general. And if you're eating fewer carbs, you're *probably* consuming fewer processed foods, too.

It doesn't really matter which of the various fad diets you follow. As long as you do what they say—and follow it with a good amount of consistency—you'll see positive results.

The problem, as I'll later explain in this book, is that it's not always so simple to just *follow the plan*. Many other things come into play, which is a lot of what the rest of the conference was about.

■ ■ ■

I went for a long run on one of the days I was there. I was training for a race, and New Orleans seemed like an interesting city to jog around. As I ran, I thought about many of the people I'd met at the conference. Folks who told me their stories about struggling with obesity all their lives.

People who were doing everything they could and still felt so awful because of how society treated them. People who probably wished they could go for a run as easily as I could, even if I am not that great at running.

It really put everything into perspective for me. Medically, I've spent a lot of my life classified as obese. But I'm still able to do a lot of things many folks can't do. I can run. I can lift weights. I don't get winded easily playing with my niece and nephew.

I am truly fortunate, even if I am often sidetracked by my own internal issues with weight bias. It's always good to reflect, I think, on the good things going on in your life. And to know that you're probably doing a lot better than you may think.

3

Marketing Your Health, or Big Wellness Takes Over

THE WELLNESS INDUSTRY

A s some point in the past few years, we stopped talking about getting healthy. Instead, we started talking about "wellness."

Throw that word into Google and you get almost half a billion results.[1] Wellness is *big money*, bringing in $30 billion in revenue in 2017.[2] It's also a popular buzzword.

In Chicago alone, I found almost one hundred businesses with "wellness" in their names, all related to some form of health care, including gyms and spas, as well as chiropractors, massage therapists, weight-loss coaches, and psychotherapists. And also a few martial arts locations, because being able to defend and attack someone is *definitely* a part of wellness.

I guess.

My big problem with the word—and I am not alone—is that it tends to be used in place of real science as a way to take your money. A meaner person would say "scam."[3] I would instead call it "a person trying to get your money through possibly deceptive means."

The reason this industry is doing so well is that it ties together nicely with something that's a big part of our lives: advertising.

But before we dive in, let me explain how a lot of advertising works and how we truly figured it out in the last one hundred years. And I'll use an oft-cited example: your bad breath.

YOUR STINKY MOUTH

In the early 1900s, people had bad breath. People had been trying to fix this for a long time, but it wasn't exactly a problem folks regularly spent time thinking about.

Enter Listerine.

The mouthwash product had been around since the 1880s, first hitting the scene as a surgical antiseptic. It was created by Jordan Lambert and named after the founding father of antiseptics, Dr. Joseph Lister.

Listerine was initially meant to clean your floors, treat your gonorrhea, and clean your feet—aka the three biggest problems of the 1800s.

It wasn't until the 1920s when Lambert's son combined *halitus*, the Latin word for "breath," and "osis," an English word that means "this sounds like something really, really medical and totally not made up," inventing the term "halitosis."[4]

And voilà, this was a "medical" term for bad breath. They repositioned bad breath as something that you should be ashamed of, and thankfully there was a cure—Listerine.

One ad from 1928 has a headline that reads, "Halitosis makes you unpopular." Then later, the same ad states: "No matter how charming you may be or how fond of you your friends are, you cannot expect them to put up with halitosis (unpleasant breath) forever."

And just like that, your self-worth is now tied to a *medical problem* that you should be *ashamed of*, and fortunately for you, there's a company that makes a product that solves this. Shame be gone!

This ad also has a fun message in the bottom-right corner, appearing to be more scientific: Sixty-eight hairdressers said that every third woman, many of them from "the wealthy classes," had bad breath. So this is a problem not just for the poors, but also the riches! Oh no!

That's how advertising works. It creates a problem that doesn't *really* exist or isn't exactly a problem, makes you feel shame for it, and then offers a solution.

The most effective ads follow the same formula: Name a problem. Shame you for having it. Offer you the fix.

This is how a lot of the wellness industry works. The core problem they push is that you are currently not well and you *deserve* to feel well, so you should pay them to make you feel well.

This leads to a lot of people who feel emptier inside, who think they can solve their problems simply by buying things, only to be out a lot of money and maybe not have their underlying problems actually fixed. Which, in turn, causes them to search for more answers, spend more money, and continue the cycle.

I'm not acting like I am somehow above this. I fall for it *all the time*. Do you know how many supplements I used to (and still!) buy, thinking they would fix my problems? (I ordered two the day after writing a section—which you are about to read!—on how supplements are bullshit. *Why did I do this?* Because someone I perceive as smart told me I should try them to see if they work. Persuasion is a helluva drug.)

The way toward health and fitness hasn't changed very much in the last one hundred years, and neither have those trying to take your money through modern-day snake oil.

SNAKE OIL—THE LITERAL AND THE FIGURATIVE

According to one study, the weight-loss industry is worth as much as $66 billion.[5] But despite all that money being spent, we aren't seeing results.

There are a few reasons for this, but here's the biggest: A lot of what's being sold doesn't work. It's just marketed well and uses suggestive language to make you *think* it's supposed to work.

I'm not calling these folks snake-oil salesmen, but let's quickly go through our nation's love affair with elixirs that people say will have results when, in actuality, they do jack shit.

SNAKE OIL GETS A BAD RAP

Real snake oil actually *worked*.

When Chinese laborers immigrated to the United States in the 1860s to work on the Transcontinental Railroad, they brought some of their ancient remedies with them. After a hard day, they would rub their muscles with an ointment made from Chinese water snake.[6]

It wasn't until almost 150 years later that a researcher discovered the snake oil contained omega-3 fatty acids, which can soothe inflammation in your muscles and joints and help cognitive function.

The problem was, what a lot of folks outside the Chinese community sold didn't even contain snakes! Now you know. And knowing is half the snake battle.

Patent- or proprietary-medicine hucksters became popular in the mid-1800s. Back then, people could say just about whatever they wanted about anything.

You could throw vinegar into a bottle, give it a cool name like Henry Jessup's Cure-All, and tell people that it could add twenty years to your life and cure your arthritis. Sometimes these remedies actually came from other cultures—notably, one made from a Native American concoction involving rattlesnakes (and the aforementioned Chinese snake oil)—but usually they were just made up.

Salespeople would travel from town to town, usually putting on a show while they hocked their wares. There would typically be a presentation during which a "random bystander" was "cured" by their "magical tonic."

People would swarm to buy it.

Patent medicine started to go the way of the codpiece by the turn of the century, especially as more American doctors decided to believe in these things called germs. And after an American newspaper published a takedown of patent medicines, showing their sellers as the con artists they were and the sometimes poisonous effects of their products, Congress passed the Pure Food and Drug Act in 1906, creating the beginnings of what would become the Food and Drug Administration.

This legislation meant that the government actually *tested* what you were saying. It was put up or shut up, and a lot of places realized, oh dang, they had to shut up. They started to put on their labels phrases such as "known as snake oil" or "for years called snake oil but does not contain snake oil."

Gives you a lot of confidence as a consumer, doesn't it? Imagine if you went to buy something today and it said, "for years called Boner Cures but does not contain any known cures for erections but is instead named after Jonathan T. Boner."

Basically, we decided you can't just lie when trying to sell something, especially if you claim it has medicinal properties.

And then everything was perfect and nobody ever lied ever again—the end.

Nope.

That hasn't stopped anyone from continuing to use slippery, meaningless words that don't mean anything but *sound* like they do.

Kind of like me calling myself an "award-winning journalist." I mean, I am an award-winning journalist, but, like, does that really make me better? Awards are arbitrary, you know? And *what* awards am I referring to? My middle school track-meet participation award? Contributing to the 2012 Pulitzer Prize for Breaking News Reporting? The Nobel?

(Two of those I have received. Guess which!)

But still—without context, words can be meaningless. Which is why lots and lots and lots of people do their best to throw words that mean nothing onto things.

Here are some words to look out for that basically *mean nothing* if you see them on packaging or in product claims:

- Acts
- Appears
- Effective
- Helps
- Is useful
- Looks
- Optimum
- Seems
- Supports
- Works

If a weight-loss product—or any other kind of product purporting to "fix" a problem—doesn't say "FDA Approved," then you should probably run away. Don't let new modern snake oil get you.

In a similar vein, when you're at the grocery store, there are some terms you may run across on food packaging that are, at best, marketing crap and, at worst, misleading and harmful. They're usually on processed foods, which is yet another reason to avoid these items. (You'll learn more about that later in this chapter.)

Because ask yourself this: If they have to *trick* you into eating it, then is it really all that good for you in the first place? Here's what to look out for:

- **Organic**—This may be a farming practice, but it doesn't really mean anything.
- **100 calories per serving**—This usually means they changed the serving size so that it's only 100 calories. The packaging may still have five servings, but each is only 100 calories. It's a way to trick you into thinking you're eating less when, in fact, you may be eating more.
- **Low fat**—This usually means a lot of sugar was added.
- **Whole grain/whole wheat**—Unless they're giving you a percentage, it could be only a tiny bit of whole grain or whole wheat and the rest is just white flour. So, basically, white bread but sold at a higher price. Look for a percentage to help you make up your mind, or check the nutritional information.
- **100 percent of your daily vitamins and minerals**—This just means they added vitamins and minerals that weren't there naturally into the food. While it's not bad, it's better if you get these vitamins and minerals from a wide variety of sources, not just one food.
- **Made with real beef**—How *much* real beef? If it doesn't say, it's probably not much.
- **Made with real fruit/vegetables**—How *much* real fruit or vegetables? And also, as opposed to what? Fake veggies?
- **Good source of [insert thing here]**—Sure, it may be fortified with this thing, but it could still contain lots of sugar and other additives.
- **No sugar added**—This just means that you're eating all the sugar that was inherently in the food, which could be a lot.
- **100 percent natural**—As opposed to unnatural, I guess? Like a vampire!
- **Part of a healthy diet**—Says who?

RED BULL'S CLASS-ACTION WINGS

Red Bull actually got sued in a class action lawsuit for its slogan "Red Bull gives you wings." Basically, a litigant who had been drinking the beverage for more than a decade argued that Red Bull's slogan was misleading, and he didn't see any increased performance, concentration, or reaction speed.

The company denied any wrongdoing and settled out of court, agreeing to put $13 million into a pool from which people who had bought the drink could claim either a $10 reimbursement or $15 worth of Red Bull products.

At the time, the company said they settled the lawsuit to avoid the litigation's cost and distraction. "However," the company wrote in a statement, "Red Bull maintains that its marketing and labeling have always been truthful and accurate and denies any and all wrongdoing or liability."[7]

I drink Red Bull. (Sugar-free only!) I never expected it to give me wings. But it just goes to show you how important a company's wording can be when explaining the benefits of their products.

MARKETING SUPERFOODS AND SUPPLEMENTS

Every other day some blog post makes the rounds, or a new study comes out, or an article runs in some publication deciding some new thing is a *"superfood."* I just googled "superfoods" and the search had more than 44 million results. By those odds, every single food is a superfood. Including things you can't eat. (Note to self: Try to make a blog post about tire rubber being a new superfood.)

Superfoods don't exist. Do you *really* think [insert random fruit, most likely with an exotic-sounding name] is going to save your life?

If that were true, don't you think your doctor would be, you know, prescribing it as medicine?

They're just foods. They usually get called "superfoods" because they contain some micronutrients that are supposed to help you. Or maybe they fight cancer. Or maybe they help your heart. The key word here being "maybe." It's *always* a "maybe," because in order for something to be truly described as being beneficial to you, at least in America, you have to, you know, prove it to the FDA.

So why do these things get called "superfoods"? The same reason lots of things suddenly become fashionable: marketing. Most likely a trade organization for that specific fruit or vegetable or meat or whatever decided to spend a lot of money promoting it. And they needed a hook to get news organizations and bloggers to write about it.

Remember *"Got Milk?"* Do you think that came out of thin air? No. It was a marketing campaign made by advertising professionals to increase milk sales for the California Milk Processor Board.[8] (It was later licensed for other dairy farmers and milk processors.)

That's the sort of thinking behind why a lot of these newly touted fruits and vegetables are deemed superfoods. Just imagine a group of ad executives sitting around and planning to drum up sales.

"What if we call it a 'superfood' and say, 'It may boost your immune system'?" they probably said at meetings somewhere. "And we'll maybe fund some studies geared toward getting an outcome we want!"

On top of that, you've got people who like reading about health-related shortcuts, especially when it comes to food. Because people like to read that sort of thing, some less-than-scrupulous news websites are definitely willing to peddle this superfood crap, because it gets eyeballs and clicks. And maybe those websites *also* sell what they're saying is good for you. What a win-win for them, huh?

If you think this is me sounding cynical, it's not. It's just the way the world works. It makes it difficult for the consumer to decide what food to buy. Can some of these products labeled as "superfoods" be good for you? Probably! I eat a few of them. But that doesn't mean I think they are going to solve all my problems or should necessarily replace my regular meals.

Because there are no shortcuts when it comes to your health. There are methods to make things easier, but if someone is promising you a shortcut, it usually means it won't work.

Don't buy into the superfood hype. Regular food will do just fine.

Addicted to supplements

As big of an appetite as we've got for supposed superfoods, America's got an even bigger hunger for dietary supplements, which is the name the food industry uses for things that are not necessarily food but that they think you should be eating. These may include fish-oil pills, vitamins, whatever. Americans spent more than $32 billion on the dang things back in 2012, which is equivalent to every man, woman, and child in the country spending $100 a month, more than the cost of most gym memberships.[9]

Supplement sales increased steadily in the past few decades after a law in the early 1990s allowed companies to sell and promote supplements as long as they were said to be "supporting" a person's health—as long as they weren't claiming to, you know, treat, prevent, or outright cure anything that's wrong with you.

Why do we take them, then?

You may already be onto me here, but there's a simple answer: marketing.

We all want to feel good. And we want to think there's an easy solution. If your doctor can prescribe some pills that make you feel better, and there are bottles of stuff near the pharmacy that say they can "support" you in various ways, well, what's the difference? A lot, actually.

My doctor, for instance, did some blood work and found my vitamin D was lacking. I live in Chicago, where the weather is legally allowed to be nice for only seventeen days a year. That means I don't go outside as much, or if I do, I cover up most of my body to protect me from the city's harsh elements and its unruly pigeons. I don't make as much vitamin D from the sun, so I need to take supplements to help with that.

Others can become iron deficient, either from their diet or from other naturally occurring things with their bodies, such as women who have heavy periods. This would be a good reason to take iron supplements. As women get older, calcium deficiency can lead to osteoporosis, so a calcium supplement may be warranted.

But unless a doctor is telling you to specifically take something, odds are it won't do anything to help you, and it may, in fact, hurt you. As an example, a 2007 study by the National Cancer Institute claims that men who took multivitamins were twice as likely to die from prostate cancer as men who didn't take multivitamins.[10]

I don't say this to scare you. I mean, I also occasionally take a multivitamin. Plus some fiber gummies. Okay, yes, you got me: I also take fish oil pills sometimes after I lift weights. Do I actually think any of these things help?

Nope. I just do them because I do them. Also because, at least for me, I think taking them is part of my process of staying on track—they've become part of my routine, if that makes sense. Wake up, eat healthy, have the multivitamin, lift weights, take the fish oil. The placebo effect is a thing.

I don't necessarily think any of them are altogether beneficial. I logically know it's kind of like throwing money down the trash chute. But I still do it, because somewhere in my brain I think that if I stop, maybe it'll mean I'll stop exercising and eating healthy.

Not to mention, what they say is in the bottle may not actually be there. In 2015, the New York Attorney General accused four big retailers of selling fraudulent supplements.[11]

That AG's office actually did DNA tests of supplements, finding that just 21 percent of the herbal supplements actually had DNA from the plants listed on the labels. Only 4 percent of the products of one large retailer—whose name is omitted here because I don't want their most-likely Arkansas based lawyers to get mad at me (hint hint)—actually showed DNA from the plants listed on their labels.

If I lied to you 96 percent of the time, what would you do? Probably not continue to believe me, right? And yet, people still buy supplements. Oftentimes because some super-ripped man or woman told you to buy them. (And guess what? They were most likely paid to say the supplements are great.)

Good supplement vendors do exist, mind you. Various websites are run by actual chemists who buy and test products of all varieties to prove they contain what the labels say they do. If you'd like to buy some supplements for whatever reason, I'd suggest seeking out those chemist-run sites that actually test different supplement brands.

That being said, you don't need supplements. Maybe the placebo effect works for you, sure, but otherwise? They don't really work. And if you properly read the labels, you'll see that they don't even actually claim they work.

The easiest way to prevent yourself from getting into this supplement trap? Don't spend money on supplements unless your doctor says you should. Here's a list of things to spend money on instead:

1. Nice shoes
2. A gift for your mom
3. A donation to your area public radio station
4. Cake ingredients (make your office a cake!)
5. 87 copies of this book

The best vitamins come from eating food, not a pill.

ANDY DOES A COSMETIC PROCEDURE

You know what else is marketed to a lot of folks? Plastic surgery and cosmetic procedures. And I was definitely led toward learning more about one specific procedure because of some random ads on the internet.

Near the end of 2017 I went into a beauty clinic. I had heard about this procedure called CoolSculpting, which is supposed to literally freeze fat cells off your body. The FDA is relatively chill about it (get it, because it's *cold*). It's been around almost a decade, and lots of studies have been done on it. And a facility that offered it was just a twenty-minute walk from my house.

I decided, for science, to check it out.

I've got a tiny bit of history with cosmetic procedures, or maybe a better term is some sort of "medically allowable body augmentation." When I was a senior in high school, my mom asked me why I never took my shirt off when I did things outside or swam in our pool.

(Yes, we had a pool in Nebraska. No, I didn't live on a farm. Yes, my high school did have corn growing a few hundred yards from it. Didn't yours?)

My fear of removing my shirt wasn't because of my weight. I was a hairy beast, like Tom Selleck except on my front *and* back. I'd been told that back hair, and shoulder hair, and even arm hair was disgusting. I don't remember who told me specifically, other than *all of popular culture ever*, but it made me not want to take my shirt off.

Oh, and I wasn't rail thin like all the other guys. One time in middle school, I was playing a basketball game with some other neighborhood kids, and when it came time to choose shirts versus skins, it was decided before I could speak that I would *definitely* be on the shirts team, otherwise it would be gross. Aren't kids *awesome*?

(Not to mention, I was raised Catholic and have all those fun issues relating to my body because of it. It's a temple, but *it is also dirty and no one should see it*.)

So my mom did what moms do and looked for a way to help. She found a place nearby that did laser hair removal. I had a consult with a doctor, my mom said it would be okay, and we would think on it. I remember the cost being something like $3,000.

That was, and remains, an insane amount of money. My family wasn't rich, but we lived comfortably, especially when compared with many others. But my parents thought three grand was a small price for their kid's self-esteem. (They're pretty awesome parents.)

At eighteen, I thought if I spent that much money to get rid of some pesky back hair, it would mean I was super vain, and that's not how people should be. I was supposed to be cool and not give a rip what others thought about me.

I also realized that, well, girls seemed to still like me despite the extra hair. I didn't get the procedure, and I'm still okay about it.

When I went in to learn about how to freeze some fat cells off my sides and stomach, I was still apprehensive. "Who does this?" I thought to myself as the technician, a nice woman in a pretty dress, walked me into an exam room. The answer: thousands of people. The technician told me she had done three thousand of these in the last eight years. And that's just her.

She had me take off my shirt and then squeezed various parts of my stomach and sides, getting an eye for how much fat was available to be frozen. Quite a bit, it turned out. It's quite strange to have some random lady squeezing your love handles and talking about how you're a "good specimen."

I left and she emailed me a quote for the procedure. It was, uh, excessive—$6,550. I didn't know it'd be that expensive, and it was ridiculous. Eighteen-year-old Andy was even more appalled. This procedure wasn't for me, I told them, and they were fine with that.

Then I changed my mind

The next few months, I ate well, I exercised regularly, and I lost a lot of weight. Then the cosmetic institute emailed me—they were having a big discount sale, would I like to come in for another exam? Sure, I thought, why not.

This time they cut their prices in half. I'd like to say it was because I had lost so much weight and they were rewarding me for a job well done, but I assume it was just a normal sales technique. Try to upsell you at the beginning, give a discount later. Like I'd gone to a shoe website, put some Nikes into my cart, then left the site without checking out, whereby they'd send me the obligatory "Oh hey, want 25 percent off?" email, like they do.

I told the clinic yes.

For science!

(And because I could probably write it off on my taxes. Past the age of thirty, the majority of what you care about are tax write-offs.)

A few weeks later, I showed up to the clinic. They took some before photos, weighed me, and had me wear a fancy robe before leading me into a room with a television and a giant machine that would be used to freeze my fat.

Now, a little more about how the procedure works: Your fat cells multiply when you gain fat, and they literally can balloon up or shrink. If you lose a bunch of weight, your fat cells don't disappear; they just get tiny. But if you start eating more calories than your body needs, those fat cells can plump right back up again. This is one reason it's easier for people who were previously overweight to gain the weight back so fast. Thanks, deflated fat cells.

Techniques like CoolSculpting help kill those excess fat cells. This isn't a weight-loss procedure—they're not taking out huge chunks of fat, similar to liposuction. It's more like they're helping you sand off some of the rough edges by getting rid of those fat cells.

If anything, I told myself, the procedure would help me get rid of some of those extra fat cells I'd gained over the years.

Andy freezes his fat

At my appointment, the technician drew some lines on my love handles for where the applicators would go, which made me feel really sexy, let me tell you. Then the applicator sucks in your fat and drops it down to minus 11 degrees Celsius, which is Canadian for 12 degrees American. The suction is pretty weak, like how I imagine a stingray would suck on a rock. (I'm no marine biologist, but I don't think they do this.)

After a short time, your skin gets numb. It really didn't hurt during the thirty-five minutes they do on each side.

While they froze my first love handle, I was texting lots of people:

"How very medical this all looks," my then-girlfriend texted after I sent her a photo.

"Ya it's medicine," I responded. "Medicine 4 hotness."

"Ya," she replied. "Sessy medicine."

You can tell a relationship is going well when you text this poorly to each other.

I sent a photo of me with the applicator on giving a thumbs-up to my mom with the caption "Getting my fat frozen off!"

She appropriately replied, "Well, I don't know what one says to that."

When the timer was up, the technician took off the applicator and started to massage the frozen area. This is when it started to sting a bit, like when you come in from the frigid cold, also known as "standard Chicago winter temperature," and your body is like, "Why did you do that to us? How dare you! We're going to make this hurt for a moment to remind you to never do it again."

After a minute, it was just numb, like your mouth after getting a filling replaced at the dentist. The technician said that'd last up to two weeks, though I got most of my feeling back after a few days. She did my other love handle, and after texting everyone else I knew with even more photos of me with my fat in a suction machine, I was done.

The procedure was costly. Let's be clear: *$2,400* was the final price tag for two separate treatments—this one and another session six weeks later. Most people who don't have book advances that they can use for research and a tax write-off may not be able to afford something like this.

And after having the procedure, I didn't immediately notice the effects. About a month later, when I was standing inside a cold building, I totally noticed where fat was no longer on my sides—they were much colder than the rest of my body. I couldn't easily tell if I looked skinnier, but others commented on it. My pants did seem to fit a bit better. But it did one thing especially well: It made me want to continue the hard work.

In the weeks that followed, I ate better. I stuck to my exercise schedule. I slept better. Just like many other things that help motivate people, getting my fat sucked and frozen was something that helped motivate me. While it may not be for everyone, it definitely had a net benefit for me.

I SHOWED MY THEN-GIRLFRIEND THIS CHAPTER AND THIS WAS HER VERBATIM RESPONSE

> beb if bad textin is a sign of goodlationships
> we should already be years married cuz we text
> v b

Translation:

> Babe, if bad texting is a sign of good relationships, we should already have been married for years because we text very bad.

HOW GYMS WORK (AND HOW THEY KINDA DON'T)

Most gyms, especially corporate chains, don't exist to make you healthier. They exist to get your money. Most couldn't care less if you ever show up. It's just more proof of how good marketing can trick you into signing up for something.

Gyms and health clubs need about ten times as many members as they can actually handle at their facility to make money.[12] Think about that: Failure is built into the basic premise of a gym.

About two-thirds of people who pay for a gym membership *never go*. I should know: I've been that person many, many times.

When I lived in Boston, I belonged to a gym in Southie. I walked past it coming home from work all the time and decided, "You know what, I should sign up!" I walked in, filled out some forms, gave them my debit card so they could charge me every month (plus the initiation fee, which was probably a hundred bucks back then), and left, feeling pretty happy about myself.

Guess how many times I went back to that gym?

Just as many times as I've dunked a basketball. Zero! (For the twelve people who thought the answer was something else, thank you for thinking I could dunk.)

I actually changed the route I walked to and from work, adding about a half mile to my commute every day, just so I could avoid feeling guilty as I walked past the gym. So, did my gym get me to exercise more? Technically, yes.

I was even paying for this gym for about three months after moving to Chicago because I was too scared to call to tell them I had moved. Do you think gyms rely on this? Yes, they do!

Just how AOL (remember AOL?) still makes a lot of money off people who've forgotten they still have and are paying for AOL accounts (LOL remember AOL?), gyms make a large chunk of change off people who've stopped going or don't remember they're paying for it. (Go make sure you're not still paying for AOL.)

Gyms are valued at around $27 billion in America, and almost $76 billion worldwide. That's a lot of money being spent for something that often doesn't work.

Why do we go?

So why do we keep doing something that doesn't work? Because gyms make it *look* like they work.

(And because if you follow a proper diet, which I explain later in this book, then the exercise *can work* to a greater extent.)

I mean, the inherent concept of a gym makes sense. It's a place where fit people go, and where people who aren't fit go to try to get more fit. If gyms didn't work, why would they continue to exist?

Let's talk about how most modern gyms are designed. You've usually got a huge area dedicated to treadmills, ellipticals, and stationary bikes. This part of the gym is usually packed. Oftentimes, gyms have entire classes dedicated to these sorts of cardio activities. They can pack thirty people into a relatively small space, get them to sweat, and get 'em out in an hour.

As you'll read in chapter 7, doing only cardio isn't enough. You have to change your diet and *maybe* do strength training—aka lift some weights.

But the strength-training part is not just scary to many. It's also cost-prohibitive.

Back to that scenario of thirty people in a relatively small space: You need just one instructor, who can keep track of everyone. Also, because they're doing cardio, less individual training needs to occur.

Not so with strength training.

Go to the free-weights part of your gym—no, not the section with machines. The area with barbells, squat racks—that spot. See how much space a single squat rack takes up? You can probably fit three treadmills in the same spot.

You can get more people in and out of your gym using less space if you focus on cardio rather than on strength training. More important, it's much more cost-effective to focus on cardio than on strength.

That's why we focus on it.

Because dollar, dollar bills, y'all.

Why should you go?

Because if you regularly go to the gym and follow a routine, any routine, you'll see results.

I talk about this later in the book, but unless you've got the cash to build a home gym for strength-based exercise, it's a good investment to join a gym and invest the time to go regularly.

Gyms work if you make them work. My gym doesn't have everything I could possibly want. But guess what? It's got the grand majority of things I need.

Your gym doesn't need to be fancy for you to succeed. If that's something you think would make you more likely to go, cool—look for that sort of gym.

But remember: Gym owners don't expect you to actually show up. Prove them wrong, get your money's worth, and get your sweat on.

DESPITE THE MONEY SPENT, WE'RE FATTER THAN EVER

The U.S. fitness industry made $30 billion in revenue in 2017, making it the most fruitful in the world. But are we any healthier?

Nope! We constantly grow more obese as a nation. Maybe that should tell you that a lot of what we're spending money on doesn't work. (Especially if it promises to get you results fast.)

FASHION AND WEIGHT LOSS

Finding good-fitting clothing as a larger person is hard. It's even harder if you're a large woman. (I don't know this from experience, obviously, but from many folks I've talked to.)

Big and tall stores are also kind of a lie. They are usually for big *or* tall people, not those of us who are large in both senses. Not to mention that every big and tall store I've been to looks like it's trying to dress men and women who are about to be on an ESPN pregame show.

As a dude, I had one place I could buy nice jeans: Eddie Bauer. I found one size that fit me great and looked nice. So I did what a lot of other large people know they have to do: I bought as many pairs as I could find.

You get used to this. You find something that works and looks good on you, and then the companies either stop making it or change it so it no longer fits like it used to.

Some companies don't even make clothes that are meant to fit larger people. Famously, Abercrombie and Fitch's brand took a hit in 2013 after some old comments of its CEO resurfaced, in which he said he didn't want "fat" or "not so cool" kids wearing its clothes.[13]

The CEO later backpedaled, saying that his company was "completely opposed to any discrimination, bullying, derogatory characterizations or other anti-social behavior." Oh, okay, dude. If that's the case, why have I never been able to find a shirt in one of your stores that fits my wide shoulders?

Some companies are starting to get it, though, as about two-thirds of Americans fall into the plus-size clothing camp. In 2018, Walmart bought the plus-size clothing brand Eloquii.

But making those clothes is smart business sense. More than half of U.S. women between the ages of eighteen and sixty-five wear a size 14 or higher.[14] (In high school, I was a cool punk rock kid and wore women's jeans. Don't judge—they looked cool, and I was an early adopter of skinny jeans. I was a size 16. Even then it was hard for me to find jeans in my size at most stores.)

For a long time, most stores sold their plus-size clothing only online, which made it harder to try on and find clothes that fit. But more companies, such as Old Navy, are starting to have those sizes in stores.

Think about when you go to most shops. The plus sizes are rarely mixed in with the "normal" size clothes. You usually have to go to another level—out of sight, out of mind—or a corner of a store to find the clothes that fit.

There's a lot of work to be done in these areas, though. Many times retailers don't reshape their clothes when they increase the size, so the sleeves, the length, and the width of the chest, among other parts, may not fit properly on a larger body. They often don't redesign clothes for different shapes but instead just increase everything at a similar rate, meaning the proportions don't always increase perfectly, which many retailers are starting to figure out.

For me, I would often find dress shirts that were the right size in my chest and shoulders, but then the sleeves were about twenty-seven inches too long, and the shirts usually drooped below my crotch. I looked like a child playing dress-up.

When I lost a lot of weight and was able to find pants in "normal" sizes again, it was insane the varieties that I could now wear. I didn't even know you had different styles of jeans! I just thought all jeans were sorta ugly but at least they covered your legs, as society requires in an office setting.

The only reason companies are starting to make better-fitting clothes for bigger people is money. They aren't doing it out of the goodness of their hearts.

But thankfully they're starting to get it, even if just a little bit. Now I no longer have to shop for just one brand of jeans. I can get all kinds!

WEIGHT-LOSS GADGETRY

Repeat after me: If it's being sold on television, it probably doesn't work.

That doesn't mean these things won't *help*. But, uh, a lot of them are silly, and you're better off spending your money elsewhere. Here's a brief overview of weight-loss gadgets:

1. Gustav Zander's fitness contraptions. This Swedish inventor made some crazy stuff, most of which looks like it should be on the set of *Fifty Shades of Grey*. Imagine a bunch of pulleys and things that spin. Nobody loses any weight, but they probably do lose a lot of their dignity.
2. Three-minute anythings. These are usually geared toward a specific part of your body, maybe your abs, or your legs, or your arms. It usually involves some kind of board, and it's supposed to get you perfectly in shape in only three minutes. Uh, no.
3. The Shake Weight. 'Nuff said.
4. Vibration belts. I don't understand how these are supposed to work—you stand while a thing shakes you? And somehow you are skinnier? Is your body supposed to just get really angry at being possibly dizzy and then you'll drop ten pounds?

5. Cigarettes. Old tobacco campaigns used to tell people that smoking cigarettes would help them lose weight. "Reach for a Lucky instead of a sweet," said one campaign in the 1920s, apparently realizing that death from possible lung cancer would mean quite a bit of weight loss indeed.

SMOKING IS STUPID

1. You don't smoke? Good for you. Keep it up.

2. You do smoke? You should quit.

3. It's one of the best things you can do for your health.

4. I mean, you picked up this book about transforming your health and teaching yourself better habits, right? You must be looking for a change.

5. Start with one that's guaranteed to make your health better: Quit smoking.

6. I know, you've heard it probably a thousand times before. But this time, make it stick. You're here to improve your health. Make this a part of it. Not to mention, it's not 1997. Nobody smokes anymore.

7. (While you're at it, drink more water.)

Also, vaping is stupid, too. Scientists invented a way to make smoking look less cool while *still* making it bad for you. Don't do it.

Look, if it's being marketed to you at all, especially if they're saying it's a shortcut, it probably doesn't work. Because there aren't any shortcuts when it comes to getting in better shape or losing weight. There's just time and effort.

How many times have you seen a commercial advertising a three-to-four-mile run? Or telling you to join a gym, any gym, and do a full-body workout three days a week? Or instead of pushing you to order a juicer, to instead eat a handful of meals with unprocessed foods every day, trying to avoid simple carbs and getting a higher dose of fats and protein?

Oh, they don't have commercials about those things on late-night television. Common sense doesn't benefit anyone who's trying to sell you a mass-produced gadget.

And finally, the models they use to show off those gizmos? I guarantee you they did not get those pecs and abs by shaking something back and forth or using a bowlike device. They went to a gym, watched what they ate, and probably were born with better genes than the rest of us.

The best health gadget? Your phone

I've tried lots of different gadgets to help me in my pursuit of a healthier body. The best one in my opinion? A smartphone.

I tried a Fitbit to track my steps. I'd always end up losing it and finding it weeks later or needing to plug it in and then forgetting it when I went for a walk. While it would push me toward walking more, it was a hassle.

But my iPhone? It can track my steps. While not perfect, it gives me a decent enough idea of my activity level to push me toward moving more.

Not only that, but during the times I've been tracking my calories, guess what I used? My iPhone, with specific apps. (MyFitness-Pal is the main app I use, as do many others, to track my caloric intake. Mind you, I don't always track my calories. Guess when I've had the most success? When I track my calories.)

When I started lifting weights, I used a notebook and pen. Then I decided to track my sets and reps on my phone using one of the various fitness trackers. It worked just fine, and there was less of a chance of me losing my notebook.

Odds are that you have a smartphone that can track your steps, eating habits, and exercise.

The only other gadget that's been helpful? My fitness watch.

It tracks my heart rate and my sleep cycle, and I can use it to track my cardio-based activities. It tries to push me toward a certain number of minutes of movement a week. (I've managed to hit those minutes every week since I bought the watch, and some weeks I've doubled or tripled the number of minutes. Hooray for me!)

Finally, the last best tech gadget? A reliable scale. I've got a fancy one that syncs with my phone. Weighing yourself every day and averaging it out over time is the best way to track your weight.

Anything else people are trying to sell you probably won't work. Save your money and join a gym that you'll go to regularly or buy some cute shoes.

Fun fact: I have bought *many gadgets* sold in infomercials. Guess how many of them I have since sold in garage sales or left on the street? *All of them.*

But wait, there's more! (No, there isn't.)

ANDY THINKS ABOUT DOING COSMETIC SURGERY

I booked an appointment with a plastic surgeon in my area after googling "Chicago plastic surgeon good." I clicked on the first result, scrolled through his website, which displayed some before and after shots, and—seeing way more boobs than I had planned to on a work computer—decided he'd be good for me. (He also happened to work out of the CoolSculpting clinic I'd visited previously, which was super convenient.)

Before my appointment, I texted my friend Stephanie:

"It would be real great if the doctor just goes 'nah you're good.'"

I imagined the doctor holding up a sign saying, TO ME, YOU ARE PERFECT.

Stephanie was a bit more levelheaded. She responded:

"Andy, they aren't going to say that. They want your money even if you have the hottest bod."

She wasn't wrong. (I do have the hottest bod.) It cost a hundred dollars just for the consult, which, of course, can be applied to any future treatments. How nice of them. (This was waived because I had already tried CoolSculpting at the same clinic.)

But because the clinic was literally down the street from me, and because I am writing a book about all this, I thought it would be good to at least talk to a medical professional. Also to learn more about why between 1997 and 2015, cosmetic surgery among people who identify as male grew by 325 percent. That's a lot more folks going under the knife.

Liposuction is the second-most-common cosmetic surgery in the United States. (It used to be number one, but recently got knocked out by breast-augmentation surgery.)[15]

It's also relatively safe—an older study showed about twenty deaths in every one hundred thousand patients who underwent liposuction between 1994 and 1998. But it's still invasive, major surgery. Complications can arise, as with any other big medical procedure.

For liposuction specifically, you can have a serious reaction to the anesthetics they use to put you under, or numb your body if you opt to be awake during the procedure. Other problems include skin infections, punctured internal organs, a fat embolism (this can kill you), and life-threatening heart and kidney problems, as well as temporary or permanent numbness in affected areas.[16]

You can also have it not work so great. You may have irregular countering, meaning your skin may be bumpy or wavy, or your physique may appear misshapen. This can happen because of unusual healing, inconsistent fat removal, or the elasticity of your skin. Instead of a symmetrical look, which is part of the goal of this surgery, you may look lopsided.

It was a relatively quick meeting, lasting less than ten minutes. The doctor was nice and affable and had a good sense of humor. First, he had me take off my shirt and show him my front and back.

No judgment. Nothing mean. He checked my abdominal muscles and said they were quite strong.

We walked through my medical history, and I told him about losing a ton of weight and keeping it off. He was kind of shocked at that and asked how I did it.

Then we talked about my goals: reducing the size of my sides and tummy.

"Even at my lowest weight," I told him, "I still had that flab."

He nodded and asked me if I had the same problem areas ten years ago. I did. The doctor explained how most men are genetically predetermined to store their fat there.

"No matter how much you run, exercise, or diet, you'll still have some there."

He wasn't saying this to push surgery on me. Far from it. He walked through the difficulties of it. First, it's expensive.

After my consult, I got a cost estimate. It would be around $8,300 for power-assisted liposuction of my abdomen and love handles, which would involve using a powered wand to vibrate my fatty tissues, breaking them up so they're easier to remove. (Another method involves using lasers to heat up the fat cells and break them apart for easier removal.) Most of that was the doctor's fee; the rest was for the cost of an anesthesiologist, the tools used, and the space for the surgery.

Most people can't afford $1,000 for an elective surgery, let alone $8,300. Now, they do have payment plans. But if you need to basically take out a loan for plastic or cosmetic surgery, maybe it's not the best idea.

The doctor strongly stressed that it's invasive surgery. He sort of rolled his eyes at other doctors' claims that it was "minimally invasive," which, he said, was bogus. It's surgery, he said, and while they can do it while you're awake, in many instances they put you under, and it's done in a hospital surgical center.

The recovery takes about two weeks, sometimes longer. All the while you have to wear a compression suit—"Like Spanx, but stronger!" he said—to help with the healing process.

"Liposuction sort of makes the areas we treat like Swiss cheese," he said. "The compression helps with swelling."

The results are also not immediate. The plastic surgeon told me it sometimes takes multiple months—sometimes up to six months—before you notice any changes. For something that's deemed a quick fix in a lot of media coverage, this was surprising.

Not to mention, he told me, if you gain weight, it'll probably end up in the same spots they removed it from. Your fat tends to accumulate in the same spots because of your genetics. It'll just go right back if you don't continue to make healthy choices.

At the end of our consult, I asked if he thought I was a good fit for liposuction. Again, he wasn't pushy. Liposuction isn't a weight-loss procedure, he said. It's for contouring your body, especially problem areas.

Losing weight on your own is always better, and something he prefers his patients to do. But for folks who have stubborn pockets of fat, liposuction can make them feel better in their clothes, which, he said, is ultimately his goal.

It's about helping the patients to feel better about themselves.

He said that in my case, he didn't know if it was the best option.

"You carry your weight quite well," he told me. "When you stand up, I could notice your love handles, but that's normal. Otherwise, you look good."

It was kind of shocking to hear that from a guy whose job is to change how people look.

I had built up this idea that plastic surgeons are kinda scummy, that they want to force these changes on your body. Maybe that's because of how they're often depicted in the media.

But this doctor was nice. Not pushy. Seemed to care about what my goals were and wasn't as interested in making a lot of money off me as he was in making sure this was the right option for me. Sometimes the marketing—including the negative images pushed onto us—doesn't live up to the hype.

4

What Is Actually *in* Food, Anyway?

OUR DIETS ONE HUNDRED YEARS AGO

What we eat today is not what our grandparents ate when they were our age. Our diets have changed drastically in the last century, and not necessarily for the better.

In fact, our diets are far different from what they used to be just fifty years ago. First, let's go through some of the bad.

More calories. The average American consumed 2,481 calories a day in 2010. (And odds are, that number has gone up since then.) That's 23 percent more than in 1970. It's also way more than most people need.[1]

If we were to look at my caloric intake if I, as a relatively healthy, tall, beefy man, did absolutely nothing except lie in bed all day binge-watching the wonderful TV show *Supernatural* (and probably peed in a bucket, let's get real here), I would need 2,700 calories a day to maintain my size.

Most people aren't as big or as muscular as me, and don't burn as many calories at rest. That means most people are consuming way more calories than they need—and that means they're gaining weight.

Here are some interesting facts about how our diets compare with the past:

Unhealthy calories. Almost half those calories (about 47 percent) come from just two groups of food: grains and flours, and oils and

61

fats. In 1970, those combined groups accounted for only 37 percent of our calories.

Those groups are mostly made up of carbohydrates, which can be helpful if you're moving around a lot and need extra energy. But as our diet changed, so did our lifestyles—we're much more sedentary than we were in 1970.

Fewer good calories overall. We're also eating less meat, dairy, fruits, and vegetables than we were in 1970. We're replacing a lot of the calories we used to get from food that is more real, more filling, and more nutritional with food that's more processed, more sugary, and with more unhealthy fats.

We drink 42 percent less milk than we did in 1970. While some naysayers dislike milk and dairy products (hello, paleo-diet enthusiasts!), milk does have a lot of relatively healthy fat and protein.

Processed foods. One study said that "ultra-processed" foods make up almost 58 percent of our total caloric intake, with almost 90 percent of that coming from added sugar.

What's an ultra-processed food? The study writers define it as:

> formulations of several ingredients which, besides salt, sugar, oils, and fats, include food substances not used in culinary preparations, in particular, flavors, colors, sweeteners, emulsifiers and other additives used to imitate sensorial qualities of unprocessed or minimally processed foods and their culinary preparations or to disguise undesirable qualities of the final product.[2]

Mmm. Scrumptious.

Processed foods aren't inherently bad, by the way. Processed foods have allowed us to feed a lot of people we normally wouldn't be able to, and for a lot less money. Not to mention that they've made it possible for food to last longer.

But the big problem is all the added sugar—which is the sugar that doesn't naturally occur in food. (We'll go into that more later.)

This sort of processed food is everywhere. But why do we eat so much more processed food now than we did before? Because we make less of our own food at home and eat out more.

Some good news. We eat double the amount of chicken now, and beef intake has fallen by more than a third. This is good because, well, chicken is delicious, but also because it takes fewer natural resources (and produces less climate-changing gases) to raise chickens than it does cattle.

OUR DIETS TODAY

Fifty years ago, it was pretty normal for a family to sit around at dinnertime and eat a meal a parent made (let's be honest, usually the mother), using relatively low-processed ingredients.

It's completely different now.

Let's look at a few numbers. The first is something the U.S. Department of Agriculture calls "food away from home," or food you eat from a restaurant or a fast-food place, or perhaps something you bought on the go at a convenience store.[3]

The other number involves "food prepared at home," which, shockingly, means food you prepare at home.

In 1970, the food-away-from-home portion of the average American's diet, in terms of how much money they spent, was 25 percent. In 1985, it was 35 percent. In 1996? More than 40 percent.

But then in 2010, the number hopped up to more than 50 percent—the first time it eclipsed the amount spent on food made in the home.

This means the majority of people are spending their money eating out, rather than on making home-cooked meals. If you're thinking, "That sounds preposterous!" first of all, wow, good fancy word usage. But second, do you really think so?

Look at your own habits. I bet you eat out a lot more than you think.

I remember when everything seemed to switch for me: my senior year of high school.

I had a car (hell yeah, 1997 Cutlass Supreme!), I had a job (hell yeah, FYE at the Southern Hills Mall!), and I had enough credits to be done with class by 1:00 p.m. (hell yeah, senior specials!).

I had the means, the method, and the time to start eating out on a regular basis. Fast food was cheap—it still is—and I could pack a few friends into my car and head somewhere for lunch. My friend Molly and I had a regular Thursday-night Taco Bell run. Just because.

That same behavior followed me into college and adulthood. Most of my diet throughout my twenties consisted of breakfast from a fast-food place, lunch from a fast-food place, and then dinner from a fast-food place.

Now, I didn't have a lot of money back then. In my mind, spending eighty dollars at once to buy groceries that could last a week or two seemed like so much more money than the six- or seven-dollar meals I could eat out.

It's a problem with how we think: short-term gain versus long-term reward. We see the smaller number, even if it's more expensive over time, and can tell ourselves it's *actually* cheaper.

We also tend to think, "Sheesh, I am just so tired and busy and have so much to do when I get home, I don't have time to make food. Might as well go get something to eat, *just this once*."

But we're habit-forming creatures. *Just this once* turns into *just for every dinner*. Then it's every other meal. Then it's every meal.

You may think this problem affects people who are poor or have limited access to healthy, more expensive options. You would be wrong.

Rich households eat out on 5.5 occasions per week, while house-

holds whose incomes are less than or equal to federal poverty guidelines eat out on 4.2 occasions a week.

Rich folks, who can generally afford the healthier options, tend
to eat out more.

WHY ALL THIS MATTERS

The food you make at home is generally healthier. This may seem
like a no-duh, but the science more or less backs this up. Even processed foods that you make at home are generally healthier than
what you get when you go out to eat.

One study showed that folks who cooked food at home consumed
fewer calories overall. Researchers found that 48 percent of study
participants who cooked dinner six to seven times a week consumed
2,164 calories a day on average, including 119 grams of sugar.[4]

Meanwhile, in that same study, 8 percent of those adults ques-
tioned cooked dinner once or less a week. Those out-of-home-eaters
consumed 2,301 total calories on average in a day. Of that, they ate
135 grams of total sugar a day.

That's 150 more calories a day in their diets, and a *lot* more sugar,
than in the diets of those who eat more home-cooked meals. You
may think that's not many extra calories, but it adds up over time—
that's equal to almost a pound's worth of calories a month.

Researchers also discovered that the folks who cooked at home
generally used healthier ingredients, relying less on frozen foods,
and were less likely to go to fast-food restaurants when they ate out.

A lot of this goes back to some of the changes in our lives. Ask
any of your friends how they are doing. I bet you every single one of
them will first answer, "Busy," and then say, "And so tired."

The main truth about being an adult is that we are all busy and
all so tired. I think this is why many of us choose faster-food options
and spend less time cooking at home.

I should know. I suck at cooking. I can barely make scrambled eggs. When I do make eggs, it's usually a big blob of stuff that, while edible, makes me think the only Beard awards I'll be winning will be related to my face.

But in my own research, guess when I was able to not only lose the most weight but also maintain that weight loss?

When I cooked my own damn food.

You may be wondering: "Andy, didn't you mention something up there about mothers and how they used to cook meals?"

I did! And that's sort of how the world used to be back in the day, sure. Then a lot of women were able to get jobs in the workplace, partially because the world became a *tiny* bit less sexist, but still: In America, at least, the role of "food maker" often falls on women in opposite-sex households, even when they are working.

Some research suggests that having more women in the workplace—as well as fewer homes with two parents, one of whom is a homemaker—has led to more fast-food purchases, even if that food is eaten at home.

I have issues with the conclusions of this research: The patriarchy isn't justification for obesity. We can all find time to make healthier food for ourselves and those we love. We just need to make sure it doesn't fall to *one person* in a household to do all the work.

(Because that's what traditional gender roles have said—women make food; men make money; *Leave It to Beaver* plays in the background. So it's almost as if some scientists are saying that we're fatter because women work more. When instead what they should be saying is *men should be helping more*.)

Research shows that a higher percentage of American men are cooking now than have in the last thirty years—43 percent.[5] They also spend more time cooking—forty-nine minutes a day—than they used to two decades ago, when they only spent forty minutes.

In comparison, forty years ago 88 percent of women cooked for 101 minutes on average every day. Now the number is 70 percent of women cooking for 71 minutes a day. That's a lot of time, but still— eating at home is overall healthier.

In chapter 9, I discuss how to find more time to devote to becoming healthier, in case you need to learn how to find the time. But meanwhile, just remember that you don't have to spend time *every* day cooking meals, especially if you live alone: Meal prep, or making a lot of meals in advance, can save you time and energy, and make it a lot easier to eat healthy.

WHAT MAKES UP OUR FOOD

Before anyone can discuss food, it's important to know what it's actually made up of.

Three things make up food—what are commonly referred to as macronutrients: protein, fat, and carbohydrates. (Alcohol is a fourth, but we're gonna ignore that for now.)

Now many of you may be going, "Uh, duh, Andy, we know what those things are!" That's awesome. You're already on your way to success! But here's the thing: I went to a decent high school and got an A in health class. I even went to the University of Nebraska— Lincoln, commonly referred to as the Harvard of the Plains. (Go Big Red!)

And yet I was twenty-nine before I finally discovered (or, perhaps, truly internalized) what these three things are. So, not everyone knows. That means it's good to go over the fundamentals before we go over the fun-dumb-mentals about food. (Do you like that pun? I just thought of it. I'm very clever.)

Let's start with the first one.

Protein, or make your body lean

Protein does a lot for your body, but the main thing it's known for is this: It's used to build muscle. Fats don't build muscle. Carbohydrates don't build muscle. Protein does.

If you were building a poke bowl, your protein would be your chicken, beans, or fish.

I won't go into all the scientific things about protein here, but another thing protein does is help make you feel full. If you're eating enough protein, and at regular intervals, it'll make you want to eat less overall. Pretty nifty.

Fats, or make your body function

Fats have gotten a bad rap over the last thirty years. Because fat is also the name for a type of body tissue we carry around, people have started to assume that anything with fat in it is therefore bad for you. That's totally bogus.

Fats help regulate your hormones, act as messengers to help protein do its job, and, quite importantly, are a major source of energy. Bet you didn't know that last part, did you?

The low-fat craze that started in the 1980s has dramatically altered the types of food available in the marketplace, and that's not exactly a good thing. You need fats to survive, and you should be eating a good amount of them.

Carbohydrates, or give your body fuel

I've saved this one for last, and for good reason. Carbohydrates are probably the biggest problem we all deal with, but they've been vilified in recent years. They're the angsty teen of the food world, hanging out in the basement and listening to sad music, looking at

Supernatural-themed Tumblr pages. (This joke will age well in five years.)

Carbohydrates are actually an essential macronutrient, but for a much different reason than protein and fats are.

Carbs are your body's fuel. Think of it this way: What's a car without gasoline? That's right—a home for skunks! No, if a car didn't have gas, it wouldn't move. Same thing for your body. You need carbs to function and survive. They also help hydrate you—hence the term carboHYDRATE.

To further this car metaphor, have you ever known a broke college student with a car? They're always keeping it running on whatever change they find under their cushions, so rarely does it have a full tank. Just like that car, your body can run without a full tank of carbs.

If you overeat this macronutrient (or any macronutrient, really), you'll end up having more than you need. And that's what ends up turning into fat on your body.

That's a quick overview, because it's time to talk about carbs some more, or specifically, the worst carb of all: sugar.

Sugar, or we're going down

Have you ever eaten food that tasted good? No? You haven't? Really? Oh, you were just pulling my chain. You're such a kidder, dear reader!

Odds are, that tasty food had sugar in it, especially if it was sweet.

Now, this is where it can get a bit complicated, as we use "sugar" to mean a few different things in the ol' food world.

The most basic building block of the carbohydrate is the sugar molecule. And depending on how many sugar molecules a carbohydrate has, your body will react differently. Complex carbs take longer for your body to digest. You get these from vegetables, beans, and whole grains.

Simple carbs are just that, easier things for your body to digest. You'll find these naturally in milk, fruit, and other unprocessed foods. But the big problem is that simple carbs are usually refined into stronger concentrates, like the sugar you pour in your coffee.

That refined sugar does something amazing to your brain. Your endorphins go insane, giving you a huge rush. It's similar to how your brain reacts when you do cocaine. (Fun fact: They're both white! And even though they can both be very dangerous to your health and are generally made in poor countries, only one is illegal! Weird how that works.)

Refined sugar is pretty powerful. And also like cocaine, it is quite addictive, is made from plants, and can be purchased in most cities. The only problem is, unlike cocaine, we've put sugar into everything. (Coke is generally only on money and pocket-sized mirrors.)

You may know this kind of sugar by a different name, though: high-fructose corn syrup. (Or as the industry is trying to rebrand it, corn sugar.) This isn't the only kind of refined sugar, but it's one of the most prevalent because it's cheap and plentiful.

Because of the low-fat craze of the 1980s and onward, food manufacturers had a dilemma on their hands. Nobody wanted to eat food that said it had a lot of fat on the label. So they remade their ingredients by taking out the fat.

But there was one huge problem: The remade food tasted like dirt.

You see, fat tastes good. There's a reason all those foods we enjoyed had it in there. So food scientists had to come up with a way that not just lowered the fat content of food but also made it tasty.

Enter our old pal: refined sugar.

You could still call something "low fat" even if it had more sugar in it than the average cookie. And when you, the consumer, who has now been told that LOW-FAT IS LIFE, ALL OTHER KINDS OF

FOODS ARE BAD, see something in your grocery that says "low fat," you snatch it up.

Only problem is, this food now has a ton more calories than it used to have on account of all that delicious white gold. (Sugar, not cocaine.) You're eating something that not only isn't healthier for you, as fats are good for your body, but that also has more calories. And it's addictive!

Isn't that fun?

HOW WE GOT HERE

So why are we using high-fructose corn syrup? Well, this kind of has to deal with economics.

Back in the day, someone decided American farmers weren't growing enough corn. So the government decided to give these farmers subsidies to grow more of it. They were basically like, "Hi, we are free-market capitalists who believe in the invisible hand of the market, but we want you to vote for us, so we're going to give you a ton of money to grow the thing you were already going to grow. Thanks!"

Now, I do not mean to demean the good corn-growing folks in the world. My college mascot is literally named after one who husks corn. (Once more, with feeling: Go Big Red!) I have family members who grow the stuff.

And for an important personal disclosure, I once sold corn out of the back of a pickup at a four-way stop outside Moville, Iowa, as a summer job after my freshman year of college. So I've definitely benefited from Big Corn. (I made enough money that summer to buy a guitar I never play anymore. It also made me realize I should study harder in school because I was never going to become a punk rock superstar.)

But what happened was, we ended up with way too much corn. Smarty-pants food-science folks came up with a few uses for all that excess: Some of it ends up as a type of gasoline, called ethanol. And a lot of the rest of it ends up as high-fructose corn syrup, which was discovered in the mid-1960s as an alternative to table sugar.

And guess what industry was looking for a cheaper kind of sugar to put into its crappy-tasting food on account of losing all those fats? Food manufacturers! A match made in food heaven.

Not to mention, we've put this stuff in *everything*. Next time you want to have some fun while you're grocery shopping, randomly take items off the rack to see if the ingredient list has high-fructose corn syrup. It's in a lot of the processed foods we consume every day—including some ketchup!

In 1970, the average American consumed 4.9 pounds of corn products a year. In 2010, it was up to 14 pounds. Back then, most of the sweeteners we consumed were made from real sugar. Guess where half of it comes from now?[6]

Corn.

Now you've got low-fat everything, but also high-sugar everything. In your attempt to eat healthier, you end up consuming more calories, feeling less full and for less time, and are more likely to have these calories stored as fat.

Check the nutritional information before buying something. If it's got a ton of carbohydrates but low fat, that usually means it's packed with those simple sugars. Put it back and get something with fat in it.

Making food addictive

Now that I've explained how sugar got into everything, think of what you want to eat right now. Like, if you could pick any food and eat it without any repercussions, what would it be?

It's probably pizza, right?

(It's pizza.)

If not, is it something filled with chocolate? Chips? Or maybe cookies?

Regardless, I bet it's something highly processed or high in sugar and fats, or both. Probably salty, too.

One study found pizza, chocolate, chips, and cookies to be among the most addictive foods out there.[7] On a scale of 1 (lowest) to 7 (highest), here's how they fared when the participants' rankings were averaged out:

- Pizza (4.01)
- Chocolate (3.73)
- Chips (3.73)
- Cookies (3.71)

How does the addictive quality compare with other foods? Well, the least addictive food out there is one that's clearly obvious. Think of the number one food you do not want right now.

I'm talking real food, something that is actually (allegedly) edible.

And you were definitely thinking of one thing.

Cucumbers.

Yes, eating a cucumber, the trashiest of all the fruits, is like chewing disgusting water. (I had to google it: According to science, cucumbers are technically fruits. But according to cooks, cucumbers are vegetables. Either way, they're gross.)

Nobody would ever become addicted to cucumbers, the French horn of the vegetable world.

(Band nerds will get that joke. If you played French horn, just assume I was making fun of a trumpet player, the instrument you *wish* you played.)

Anywho, the science agrees with me: On that same scale of 1 to 7, with 1 being the least addictive:

- Cucumbers (1.53)
- Carrots (1.60)
- Beans with no sauce (1.63)
- Apples (1.66)

As for the addictive food, that's not an accident. Your body is made to want those kinds of foods. In many cases, food is engineered by scientists to be hyperpalatable—that is, made in such a way that it surpasses traditional food in terms of how it makes your brain super happy.

They're typically pumped with fat, sugar, food additives, and other flavors not found in nature. This is highly intentional.[8]

Consider Taco Bell's Doritos Locos Taco. If you need to go to your nearest combination Pizza Hut and Taco Bell to buy one for an investigation, I can wait.

It's crunchy, given its shell as well as the lettuce. It has salt in its seasoning. It has fat in its cheese as well as its shell.

And it goes down quick and easy, thanks to its "taco jacket" (yes, they call it that), which is also sometimes called a "holster." Because it's like a gun of flavor into your mouth.

Within ten weeks of its debut in 2012, this product was the most successful food Taco Bell had ever launched in the company's fifty-year history. They sold 100 million tacos during that time.[9] The tacos were offered for only a short time, but still, same formula: easy to eat, salty, crunchy, and full of fat.[10]

In comparison, McDonald's took eighteen years to sell 100 million burgers.

But this wasn't an accident. The food combined something that was already hyperpalatable—Doritos!—and mixed it with something in the same category: Taco Bell tacos!

And its bright packaging makes you crave it even more.

In 2018, guess what new product Taco Bell launched that dethroned its Locos Tacos?

French fries with nacho cheese sauce.

Look at most new fast foods that come out. They follow that formula. The code has been unlocked. Food scientists know how to get you hooked.

Which makes me wonder: We decide *some* addictive substances, such as opioids, should have safeguards around them. You need a prescription to get them. Or at least you need more warning before you start taking them.

Why are we allowing our food supply to be turned into something more addictive than hard drugs? (And, according to mortality rates, heart disease is one of the biggest killers in America. So, one *could argue,* these kinds of addictive, unhealthy foods are killing more people than the big bad illegal scary drugs that we need a war on.)

Many processed foods are made to be addictive by scientists who earn more money than most journalists writing books about them. Natural food isn't anywhere near as addictive—and it's healthier for you!

So, while you should be eating more fruits and vegetables, understand that if you find that difficult to do, it's because you're addicted to the unhealthy stuff.

Fun fact: If you work hard enough, all pizzas can be personal.

NIGHTMARE FUEL

Burger King launched a Halloween-themed burger in 2018 that they said was clinically proven to give you nightmares.

The company claimed a test showed that after people ate the Nightmare King—a burger with a quarter pound of beef, a chicken fillet, bacon, cheese, and mayonnaise—they suffered nightmares 3.5 times more than the average person.[11]

Oh, did I mention the bun is green? Because that screams delicious. (Or probably to your brain it screams, "ROTTEN FOOD FULL OF BACTERIA," which some other scientists say could be the reason it causes stress-induced nightmares.)

Of course Burger King didn't share the study publicly—perhaps it's too spooky? But if we're taking the company at their word, that means they made a sandwich so bad that it affects not only your body in terrible ways (it's got more than a thousand calories) but also your mind.

Now you've got another reason to make your way toward healthier choices: protecting your dreams.

ALL CALORIES AREN'T EQUAL (OR ARE THEY?)

What's a calorie?

Unless you remember basic high school chemistry (or you googled it after I asked), most of us don't even know what that is. It's just a thing that's put on food labels.

If you eat too many, you gain weight. Eat fewer, you lose weight. It's some sort of magical word that decides on your body's composition, right?

Not really.

A calorie is this: the energy needed to raise the temperature of a gram of water by 1 degree Celsius, or 33.8 degrees in Freedom Units. (Although, to be super technical, because someone who likes to email authors to prove they're wrong will email me to prove me wrong if I don't say this, scientists now usually define a calorie as the energy needed to raise the heat of 1 gram of water approximately 4.2 joules.)

There! Now it's perfectly cleared up for you, right?

Probably not. Let me clear it up.

So, that's what is referred to as a "small calorie," with a little "c."

What you see on a food label is actually a *kilo*calorie, which is equivalent to 1,000 small calories.

But because scientists love to make things easy for us to understand, we call a kilocalorie a Calorie. Big "C," not little "c."

Then, because we are lazy, we usually just say "calorie." With a small "c."

Making it even easier to understand.

Because science.

Look: It's just a unit of measurement. It's not a real *thing*. But because we spend so much time talking about them, we need to dive into what they are.

WHY WE COUNT CALORIES

You can attribute our current method of measuring calories to Wilbur O. Atwater, an American chemist born in 1844 who studied metabolism and human nutrition and definitely had a name straight out of 1844.

He also had a severe mustache, because it was the 1800s and no one would trust your scientific experiments unless your facial hair was impressive.

Atwater discovered that a gram of fat burned about 9 calories, while a gram of protein and a gram of carbohydrates burned 4 calories. This is all according to the previously explained caloric unit of measurement.

Think of it this way: This is like trying to determine how far a gallon of gas will go. Different kinds of gas work a little bit better or worse in the engine. Similarly, so do the macronutrients—they burn differently.

This is why a Snickers bar, which has 11 grams of fat (99 calories), 28 grams of carbs (112 calories), and 3 grams of protein (12 calories!), adds up to 223 calories. (Yet the label says 215. Because science?)

Anywho, this was decided on as the way for us to measure the calories in our food—that these numbers are inflexible and will remain this way forever, that each macronutrient perfectly corresponds to everyone's body burning exactly that many calories. And it's been perfect ever since Mr. Big Mustache figured it out. Right?

(Spoiler alert: Wrong.)

Calories aren't equal

Part of the problem with Atwater's method of food measurement is we don't deal with every calorie the same way. You don't absorb every part of the food you eat. And also, every person—depending on what's in their gut bacteria and other health factors that are unique to each individual—deals with calories differently.

One clear example of this is in squirrel food—or nuts, as you might call it. In 2008, researchers published a study showing that almonds had 20 percent fewer calories than what would be predicted using Atwater's system.[12]

One study found that pistachios (researchers love themselves some nuts) had 5 percent fewer than their guesstimated calories.[13] The reason for this? If someone eats pistachios whole—as opposed to processed, as in peanut butter—more fat ends up in their toilet instead of getting digested.

Also, your mom was right: You *should* chew your food. This same study found that the more you chomp, the more food you actually absorb. (I've yet to discover whether this means if I barely chew cookies that the calories don't count.)

When it comes to nuts, this study found that a large amount of their fat is stored inside their nutty cell walls. If those walls don't get broken down by chewing, then they may flow through your body without your body absorbing the oils inside them.

Calories make you feel different

You can do this experiment yourself. Eat two Snickers bars and then see how you feel in an hour. Probably a bit sluggish. Maybe you were hyper for a minute and then you crashed?

That's because what you ate were primarily carbohydrates in the form of sugar, along with some fats. That combination will lead to your having an insulin spike, which will later drop, causing that sleepy feeling.

(I am not bashing Snickers, by the way. It's the best candy out there, after a Twin Bing, which is a Sioux City–area delicacy. Please, Palmer Candy Company, sponsor me, even if your amazing candy does look like a dog turd.)

Now, wait a few hours, then cook yourself some vegetables—a few cups of broccoli, cauliflower, or spinach. Add a roasted chicken breast, some cheese, and perhaps a handful of plain almonds.

How do you feel after that? You *should* feel full. Not to mention, your energy levels should stay consistent for the next few hours, until your next meal.

That's because you not only ate healthier food—SHOCKER: Candy isn't that healthy for you—but the macronutrients in that food were much more conducive to giving you energy, making you feel full, and ensuring that your insulin levels don't suddenly spike and then fall.

Wait, but *are* calories equal?

There was a story about a decade ago—a college professor in Kansas ate mostly junk food for ten weeks to prove that all calories are equal. This professor of human nutrition lost twenty-seven pounds, just by eating Twinkies, Little Debbie snacks, Doritos, Oreos—all those tasty things that are probably making you crave them right now.[14]

Damn you, Doritos, and your all-powerful crunch and mouth-feel.

Anywho, the professor lost the weight because he limited his caloric intake to about 800 fewer calories than he needed a day. He also did blood work at the end, showing him to be relatively healthy.

The professor *did* drink a protein shake, ate healthy vegetables regularly, and took a multivitamin. So it wasn't junk food only.

Does this mean you should try it? Of course not. (The professor even said so, as did other health experts at the time.) The professor was only moderately overweight to begin with and had an active lifestyle.

Just because this form of eating and weight loss works for one person doesn't mean it'll work for others. Or that it's sustainable. Especially for those who already have issues with overeating or making less-than-great choices when it comes to food.

The science is clear: If you eat healthier food, your body uses it better. It makes you feel better. And it can help regulate your mood, keep hunger pains at bay, and give you the energy you need.

While the amount of calories you eat is important, the type of calories you eat also matters.

LOWERING YOUR GLYCEMIC LOAD

Your body is good at dealing with whatever you throw down your gullet. The problem is, what you're noshing on may affect your blood sugar.

If your body can easily turn something you consume into glucose—the sugar your body uses for energy—then that can lead to an insulin spike. Ever get super hyper from eating something full of sugar? That's this in effect.

Then you usually have a crash, when you feel low-energy and

sluggish as your blood sugar drops and gets closer to normal. This can lead to overeating, because your brain thinks you're now somehow in desperate need of energy.

Insulin spikes like this can cause you to store that extra energy as fat. While it's not the *main* culprit of adding extra body fat— that's simply from consuming more calories than you need in general—it can still increase it.

That's why you should focus on eating food with low glycemic loads: whole grains, fruits, veggies without starch, and legumes. Eat fewer things with high glycemic loads, such as white rice, white bread, potatoes, and other carb-heavy foods.

And, of course, those foods with the highest glycemic loads? Sugary foods like soft drinks, candy, and cake? Try not to make them the entirety of your diet. (You may already know that, but, hey, now I'm saying it again. For science.)

ALCOHOL!

As with everything in life, moderation is key. And even if you've got a lot of your food intake under control, there's another area that people forget about on their road to a healthier body: alcohol.

One survey says 86 percent of people eighteen or older said they drank at some point in their life, with 70 percent saying they drank in the past year, and 56 percent in the past month.[15]

The same survey said that almost 27 percent of those in the same age range binge-drank in the previous month, with 7 percent saying that they "engaged in heavy alcohol use" in the previous month.

This is not me preaching that alcohol is bad. Or saying you must stop drinking your Miller High Life. Or that IPAs are bad. (They actually are.) But just as sugary drinks aren't that great for you, booze, especially beer, has some similar effects.

Again: I am not advocating for everyone to become a teetotaler. Think about this from a calories-in, calories-out perspective.

One beer has about 150 calories. That may not seem like a lot, but that's just in a single a can of beer. If you're out at a bar and you get a tall boy or a large stein, it's probably closer to 20 ounces, which is closer to 250 calories. That's like drinking an entire candy bar— only if the candy bar also made you think you were the best dancer at every wedding.

Those calories can add up. If you just have a few beers after work, you may be having an extra 400 to 500 calories a day.

Even if you've got your food consumption in check, or you're exercising to help burn off some extra calories, chugging a few beers on occasion will negate some of that work.

But what about liquor? If you're drinking whiskey, or vodka, or, heaven forbid, straight shots of gin, you're doing a bit better in terms of calories. They have about half what a beer does, and usually have a similar alcohol content.

The problem with these liquors, though, is that many people like mixed drinks. Throw in some Red Bull or a Coke, and you may have a tasty beverage, but you've just potentially quadrupled the number of calories you're ingesting because of the sugar in the mixers. Again, it adds up. Not to mention, spirits will get you drunk a lot faster, which can lead to all sorts of other issues. (See: terrible dancing.)

But what about wine? A glass of red wine has about 125 calories. That's quite a bit, except the good news is that wine has substantially fewer carbs than beer does. So with a glass of wine, you're ingesting about one-fourth of the carbs while getting about the same level of alcohol that you'd get in a bottle of beer.

Wine has the same issue that other alcoholic drinks do, though: Those calories can add up. One glass of wine after dinner probably won't hurt you. But two? That's like having an extra candy bar's worth of calories. If you drink that amount regularly, consider doing something to offset the calories, or change how often you're imbibing that vino.

AN EVEN BIGGER PROBLEM

There's a bigger problem when it comes to drinking alcohol, one that happened to me constantly: the alco-hungries. Yes, this is a real term that everyone says and not one I just made up for this book. No, *you're* lying.

The alco-hungries is that part of you that decides, after you've had a few drinks, that you now need a few slices of pizza. Or maybe seventeen tacos. And two orders of chicken pad thai. (A restaurant that can deliver all these would make a killing.) Now your simple night out has ended up with you consuming the entirety of all the food in your town and probably undoing all the hard work from your entire week of diet and exercise.

On top of that, your body can't store alcohol. That means as soon as you drink it, your body prioritizes metabolizing it over anything else you've consumed, which means whatever food you're eating while drinking is more likely to be stored as fat. Alcohol impacts your ability to absorb nutrients from your food as well, which is just another kick in the pants.

I spent a lot of my twenties giving in to the alco-hungries. For instance, in Boston I used to live by a place that was open until 2:00 a.m. that served Mexican *and* Chinese food—the greatest combination ever. I ordered many gigantic burritos with sides of crab rangoon. Not to mention, they delivered, allowing me to exercise even *less*.

I think a lot of my weight gain came from the food I ate during and after my nights of drinking, not necessarily the drinking itself. And then the next day, even if I had told myself, "I'm going to eat healthy this week!" I would feel like I had thrown it all away because of my food intake the day before, and feel like it was all ruined anyway, so I might as well have whatever I wanted the next day. Thus leading to more food and more food and more food.

Not to mention, do you know how hard it is to exercise hungover? Like, you know how much you hate going to work with a hangover? Imagine how hard it is to head to the gym with a pounding headache, all dehydrated and sweating beer through your pores. Smelling like a brewery on the treadmill and everything!

If you're having struggles losing weight but are eating well and exercising regularly, take a look at your alcohol intake. I'm not saying you should give it up entirely, even though, as of this writing, I haven't boozed it up in more than five years. It's working for me and has definitely helped me with my weight and exercise goals.

A lot of my friends with fitness goals—from runners to power lifters to bodybuilders to just regular people trying to stay in good shape—have severely cut down or stopped their alcohol intake, too. It's not weird to take a break from drinking if you're focusing on your health.

If you drink regularly, even if it's not that much, it adds up faster than you think. Try cutting back and see what happens. Drink light beer. Have some liquor without mixers. And please, whatever you do, don't drink IPAs. Because they're trash.

5

Your Body, Explained

HOMEOSTASIS ISN'T ALWAYS YOUR HOMIE

Here's a little secret your body never told you: It wants you to be big.

You see, despite the amazing art we've made as a species (*Die Hard*), the wonderful literature we've created (the book that *Die Hard* is based on), and the amazing music we've invented (the soundtrack to *Die Hard*), we are actually all just a bunch of animals. We are born, we grow, then we die.

But along the way, our bodies are constantly trying to do the same thing: stay alive. (Cue the Bee Gees, who were, sadly, not featured in *Die Hard*.)

It's this little thing called homeostasis. With any changes you make to yourself, your body is forced to adapt. If you run a lot, your body's like, "Oh crap, I guess we're a runner now?" and you get better at running. If you don't drink enough water, your body freaks out and yearns for H_2O. And if you eat more than your body needs, it stores all the excess.

This isn't inherently bad. It's just how your body is.

That extra weight that you're storing—whether it be from muscle, fat, or just superheavy bones—is intended to keep you alive.

Think back for a bit to when we were a species that did not have amazing things to watch on our television at the flick of a button

(*Die Hard*). Back in the age before writing, when we were living off the land as hunter-gatherers.

Back when our food was scarce, if you encountered a bunch of it, your body would be so happy and excited. "Hooray!" your body would say. "We don't know when the next time we'll find a bunch of food will be, so instead of wasting this mastodon meat and pooping it out, let's store some of it on our bodies!" Of course, your body *probably* didn't say this in English; you probably grunted. (Give me some artistic license here, people.)

That's where your fat comes from. It's because your body is constantly afraid that your next meal may not come for a while. Now, this kind of behavior definitely made sense tens of thousands of years ago, when the only way we ate was when we used pointy sticks to take down beasts. You had to work hard for your food, you moved a lot during the day (and night), and you didn't eat that often altogether.

And now look at us. Food, at least in the Western world, is plentiful and cheap. (Don't make a "it grows on trees" joke here, Andy. Just don't do it.) We don't have to move as much as a society to get those calories and nutrients. I can literally tap my phone four times and get a burrito delivered to my home. (The future is now!)

So when we eat food, it tends to stick to us. Unless we give it a reason not to.

That's the first basic thing you need to understand about your body. But there's much more.

CALORIES IN, CALORIES OUT?

The science is simple: If you move more, you burn more calories. If your body has more muscle, you burn more calories. Exercise is one way to move more and build (or maintain) muscle mass.

This is the basic concept you may have heard a thousand times before of "calories in, calories out." That if you eat less, or use exercise to use more calories than your body needs, you lose weight.

So you should exercise, right?

It's not *entirely* that easy. Because there are so many different ways to exercise. Which is the right one? What if you choose the *wrong* one? Are you forever doomed?

First of all, let's get a few things out of the way (and yes, I first typed "way" as "weigh" because I am smart):

1. **Exercise alone won't make you lose weight.** You lose weight primarily through your diet. Exercise can *help* you lose weight. But getting your diet under control is the most important thing you can do. The old saying about how abs are made in the kitchen is true. (But really, getting abs should be no one's goal, as I explain later.)

2. **You can't pick a wrong exercise.** One study of people's exercise habits showed that just slow-walking ten minutes a day could increase your fitness level by about 3.8 percent.[1] If you do twenty minutes a day, it's about 6.7 percent. That means if you do barely any exercise, even just a slow walk, you'll see positive effects in your body. Therefore, any exercise you do is the right kind.

3. **Different goals mean different kinds of exercise.** If you want to get better at running, you should be running more. If you want to get stronger, you should be lifting more. It's fine to do a mix of both, or do a group fitness class, or climb rocks, or hike, whatever. Just find something, learn how to do it, and then do it.

4. **Sitting all day is bad for you.** Study after study shows this. Break your day up by moving around every hour. Exercise alone can't fix what happens by sitting for sixteen hours a day.

5. **You need to change your relationship with exercise from your *to-do* list to your *want-to-do* list.** Find something that's fun, that you like to do, and that isn't hell on earth. Make sure you try a few different things.

EVOLUTION AND YOUR BELLY FAT

Your body is the way it is partially because of evolution. Whatever worked best, in a genetic sense, got passed down to the next generation because they survived. If you had a way of storing excess energy in the form of fat, you'd be more likely to survive when food was scarce.

Humans have been hunter-gatherers for the majority of our time on this planet. We had to move a lot to find food, either through hunting animals or gathering plants, searching for food wherever we could. Our evolutionary needs haven't yet caught up with our modern lifestyles. Or, to quote Garabed Eknoyan, MD, of Baylor College of Medicine:

"This ability to store surplus fat from the least possible amount of food intake may have made the difference between life and death, not only for the individual but also—more importantly— for the species. Those who could store fat easily had an evolutionary advantage in the harsh environment of early hunters and gatherers."

HUNGRY LIKE THE WOLF

Your body produces many kinds of hormones. Some regulate your growth or your metabolism, and some make you bald. (I have a lot of that last one.) But your body also has two bastard hormones that do something else: They make you hungry.

These hormones are called ghrelin and leptin, and for the rest of this chapter, we're going to combine them into one word, because it's what they really are: "gremlins."

YOUR APPETITE HORMONES ARE CONTROLLING YOUR LIFE

Ghrelin is produced in your gut and tells your brain you need to eat more. It's the hormone that pushes you to seek more food, to eat more calories, and then store it as fat. Studies have shown when ghrelin levels are increased in people, they tend to eat more than those whose levels aren't, regardless of your size.[2]

Meanwhile, the hormone leptin tells you how *full* you feel. If your leptin level is high, you think you've had enough food.

When you restrict your calories, ghrelin goes up and leptin drops. This means you're not only hungrier but you also feel less full overall. What a treat for anyone trying to lose weight, right?

These punks. They're part of the reason it's so difficult to lose weight.

You ever go a few days when you're eating well, not overeating, just feeling good about your food intake? And then suddenly, out of nowhere, you get this urge:

FEED. ME.

NOW.

MUST EAT. GIVE. ME. FOOD.

That is your gremlin hormones yelling at you. They want food, and they make your body go into overdrive, thinking you're starving. If you lower the amount of food you regularly eat, they start to get out of whack, and scream at you, as if something's wrong.

These hormones aren't all bad. They're what help you realize you need food, so you don't accidentally forget to eat. They regulate your appetite, letting you know when you've had enough and when it's time to start thinking about a meal.

Studies show a person who's lost a substantial amount of weight will have higher average levels of the gremlins than someone who has never been overweight. What this means is, if you've once been fat, then lost a bunch of weight, your body's appetite function is more likely to go, "OH MY GOD! FEED ME NOW."

Yes, it's a bunch of crap. Thanks, genetics!

And yes, it's another reason why the yo-yo diet effect occurs. This is when you lose some weight, let's say twenty pounds (hooray—go you!). And then you gain thirty pounds back. (Oh no, what happened?)

This isn't because your willpower failed. It's because the appetite gremlins are screaming in your ear, telling you to eat more and more. So you overeat and gain enough weight so that you're not only back where you started but usually a few pounds heavier.

It's as if you have two screaming drill sergeants in your brain, telling you that you're starving and you need to eat. This is why you may have weeks of great habits and then suddenly you have the strongest urge to eat everything in sight. Drill sergeants can be a bit demanding like that.

This is one of the biggest problems of losing weight that I've found. You do well, and then your appetite goes into overdrive, and you can't help yourself. For me, I call this the "pizza sads." I'll get to a place where I've eaten great all week, going to bed a little hungrier than I'm used to, exercising, feeling good.

But then on a Friday or Saturday, it strikes. My appetite gets out of control, and I reflexively order a pizza. Or two. And then I eat them. *All of them.*

All that hard work, down the drain. (Or so you think.) My appetite hormones are happy, though, because they think I've done what

I am supposed to do. It becomes a cycle—one that can be hard to break.

Thankfully, for those who may be having issues with their appetite, there are some medical solutions. More than a few medications exist (none of which I've tried) that help suppress your appetite. Unlike diet pills, which are basically just a form of legalized meth, these drugs help regulate your hormones. Your gremlins get back in line with where they should be. Instead of thinking, "FEED ME, FEED ME," your body thinks, "HOORAY—I AM FULL."

Medication makes it easier for some people. And you shouldn't feel bad if you decide to talk to your doctor and go this route. Your body is fighting against you. So you should fight back.

Studies have shown that folks who were undernourished growing up—or even while they were in the womb—are more likely to become obese as they get older. Some call it the double burden of malnutrition. Overweight mothers make their children predisposed to also becoming overweight. Rapid weight gain earlier in life may also lead to lifelong battles with obesity.

And with about two-thirds of the U.S. population being overweight, that's getting passed on to children, who start this cycle early. Nearly one in five kids between the ages of six and nineteen is obese, a number that's tripled since the 1970s, according to the Centers for Disease Control and Prevention.[3] It's like kids are running a race against obesity, and they're forced to wear concrete shoes from birth.

Overweight people can also be undernourished. You can still have an excess amount of body fat, as deemed by health standards, and be deficient in the vitamins and nutrients your body needs to function.

Basically, unless you were one of the lucky minority who managed to maintain a healthy body weight their entire life with lower-than-average body fat, you're going to struggle with your size somehow.

That's the secret they don't tell you when they're trying to sell some new weight-loss plan: Your body wants to stay the same. And if you've been bigger for a long time, it's gotten used to it.

And changing your body is going to be difficult. But it *is* doable. Just perhaps not in the way you think.

ANDY VISITS HIS DOCTOR

Before embarking on a journey about weight loss, I did a thing I probably should have done years ago: I went to talk to my doctor.

As a quick reminder: I managed to lose a ton of weight altogether without the help of medical professionals. I also had no clue what my baselines were, in terms of my blood work and blood pressure. So I went to my doctor for a yearly physical and to get some of these tests done.

I also told him what I was doing: writing a book about fitness, weight loss, and why it's so damn hard to lose weight. He nodded and started some tests.

My blood pressure was great, and my eventual blood work would show that everything—except my testosterone levels—was also great (more on this later in this chapter). He then asked me what my plans were for the book.

"Well, *for science,* I gained thirty pounds, and I plan on losing it all, just so I can write about the process."

He thought about it for a second and then spoke. "You should lose more."

"More?" I asked. "Back when I was two hundred and fifteen pounds, I was pretty skinny. That's about where I want to end up."

My doctor shook his head. "You're currently considered obese." He showed me a chart listing something called the body mass index

(BMI), which calculates a number based on your height and weight. It said that I was obese, at six foot two and 250 pounds.

I would actually have to lose eighteen pounds just to be considered overweight. I looked at him. "Uh, I just ran a 10K a few months ago, I'm kind of strong because I lift weights, and you just said everything else about me shows I'm in good health."

"But you're obese," he said. "So you need to lose even more weight than you intended to be healthy."

I think if most people looked at me, they'd think I look like the "average chunky, tall American." While I definitely see a worse version of myself in the mirror than other people do, I didn't necessarily consider myself *that* fat.

For a six-two person, an ideal weight is considered to be between 148 and 193 pounds. Dear reader: I was five foot ten and 175 pounds in sixth grade. I haven't been near 193 pounds since eighth grade, when I topped out at my current height. (My mom said back then, when I was an obvious giant, that someday everyone would catch up with me. I'm still waiting on that, Mom.)

I've always been a big guy. I just carry more weight in general. Always have. Probably always will.

My doctor told me that the BMI isn't the best indicator for health, especially if you're more muscular, but it's a good start for most people. It doesn't consider muscle mass, or people who just tend to be broader than others.

So I asked, "Why use that as a tool then?"

He shrugged, said it was the best they had. (Dear reader: Your BMI does not define you. Arnold Schwarzenegger's BMI, for instance, when he was winning bodybuilding competitions left and right, would show that he was obese, too.)

My doctor slapped me on the knee and smiled. "It's okay! You're just a really healthy big guy."

Great start to my weight-loss experiment, Doc.

MY OWN GENE RESEARCH

At a DNA level, we change too slowly over time for our genes to have as much of an impact on worldwide obesity rates. But they do play a factor in why we're so big.

I decided to take a look at my own genes to see what I could figure out from them and whether they'd give me any insights into my body. (Mostly I wanted to see if I had any genes that made me predisposed to being fatter.)

The Human Genome Project is what made a lot of this possible. It was the largest collaborative biological project in the world, funded by the U.S. government and other organizations worldwide from 1990 to 2003. It was supposed to cost $3 billion but ended being a little cheaper.

This work, as well as increases in technology over the years, has led to DNA sequencing becoming much cheaper—for instance, none of us has to pay $3 billion—and faster, while also becoming more accurate.

In case you don't know what DNA is, think of your genetic makeup as an instructional manual with millions of individual letters. If on page 174 there's a certain letter—let's say "Z"—that could mean you're more likely to be lactose intolerant. But if the letter is "F," you're less likely.

Scientists use faster methods these days, in which, instead of searching for individual letters, they check more for the *"sentences"* on those instruction manuals. That's what helps give them a more accurate view of what could possibly be happening with your body, or what could be in store for your future.

Let's look at my genes

To do my own research, I first sent in my DNA to Ancestry.com. It's a simple process—you spit into a tube, close it up, and mail it out. A month or two later, you get some results. And this fact may be incredibly shocking to those of you who've seen my author photo.

I am incredibly white.

Like, super Caucasian.

I'm 61 percent from Ireland and Scotland, 38 percent from England, Wales, and northwestern Europe. That remaining 1 percent? Swedish!

Like I said, *white as all hell.*

What does that mean? For one, studies show that obesity is much more prevalent among racial minorities than white folks.[4] White people have a 26.6 percent prevalence of being obese, while for Latinx people it's 30.6 percent, and black people it's 37.6 percent.

Does this mean the genes associated with your skin color mean you're more likely to be larger? Not necessarily. A lot of issues tie into your chances of becoming obese, including education level and wealth level. And systemic issues push people of color to be less educated, have less wealth, and often live in areas that have fewer readily available healthy food options.

What this means is that those with my percentage of mega-whiteness typically have a lower chance of becoming obese than those of other races in America. (Still happened to me, though!)

I also found a lot of second cousins I didn't know about. Thanks, Ancestry.com!

The second place I took my DNA to was a company called Fitness-Genes. They purport to be able to not only give you some basic ideas of how you should be exercising based on your genes but also give you tips on what you should be eating and drinking.

That's quite a big claim to make. Again I hocked a bunch of spit into a tube and sent it off to be tested. While waiting, I looked more into what folks say about these testing methods.

The Federal Trade Commission has said that people should be skeptical about genetic tests like this:

"The results of genetic tests are not always 'yes or no' for the presence or the risk for developing disease, which make interpretations and explanations difficult."[5]

The FTC goes on to say that many issues arise from environmental factors in combination with genes and that health care experts are only beginning to understand all these issues.

FitnessGenes is pretty upfront about that, saying the results they get aren't "black and white," nor do they consider themselves a disease-predicting DNA service.

Instead, they're more interested in how your genes impact diet, exercise performance, and overall fitness, and they use peer-reviewed research to make *interpretations* based on your genes.

Basically, they test your genes and provide you with modern research about those genes, giving you an idea of what the studies out there say. It's up to you to decide what to do with that information.

The FDA toes a similar line, saying that both it and Centers for Disease Control *"know of no valid scientific studies showing that genetic tests can be used safely or effectively to recommend nutritional choices."*

Well that's fun to read, especially after I shelled out $259 to run these tests.

The FitnessGenes website counters that what they think the FDA is trying to say is there aren't any recorded studies showing a DNA company's customers benefiting in the long run from nutritional recommendations. The FDA is saying that's hard to do because the science—and these companies—has been around for only a short time, so no large-scale studies could be done.

FitnessGenes also says they collaborate with different universities and research groups and get feedback from customers. They hope to have academic publications in the future.

That's fair. But as with anything, it's how you use it.

It's important to note that in 2013, the FDA ordered another DNA testing company, 23andMe, to halt sales of its test kits because the governmental agency said the company was claiming it could alert customers about diseases they were at risk for or currently carried without getting clearance or approval from regulators.[6]

This is still kind of a squishy area for science. I wasn't planning on using the data as something to completely change my life. But I did think it'd be interesting to discover what it had to say.

Six weeks later, I got the email notification that my results were ready while I was en route to the gym. I had to wait until after I lifted weights—perhaps I was lifting them "incorrectly," according to my DNA?—and I couldn't wait to find out what I was doing right, or wrong, according to what evolution hath wrought upon my body.

After having to reset my password for the website umpteen times, I started reading through what it had to offer me.

My genes and lifestyle

Let's start with my lifestyle summaries. On the whole, most of what the data told me just seems like good advice in general.

- I may not have an increased preference for sweet snacks. This is true—I'm not exactly one to opt into a candy bar, at least not these days.

- I'm less likely to be hungry between meals. This is also quite true. Ever since I stopped working in a downtown office that had vending machines and snacks all over, I don't eat as much between meals.

- I should shoot for a lot of sleep because my circadian rhythm may be suboptimal, which means my sleep is crappier. (My tracking watch and overall daily experience seem to correlate with this.) I should also avoid exercise near bedtime and bright lights (like from a phone) before trying to sleep. Standard advice.

■ I need more magnesium than most when training. Bodybuilding forums are always talking about magnesium, which some say can improve sleep, help you poop, and strengthen your bones, so that's nothing new.

■ I have a faster caffeine metabolism than most, so I shouldn't use it as something to get me going, but instead as something to enjoy, because its normal benefit—stimulation—doesn't affect me as much as it does others, plus it leaves my body faster. This I've noticed—I rarely get the jitters after having a lot of caffeine. But I was told by the gene report that I should still avoid it four hours before bedtime. Duh.

■ The Mediterranean diet could be helpful for me, but my genes don't indicate specifically that I should favor it.

Nothing mind-blowing here, but a few things did ring true to what I've experienced—not so much helpful as it is a confirmation bias, I told myself, where I see answers that seem to confirm my preexisting opinions.

Next came nutrition.

■ I can tolerate foods with a high glycemic load and not see too many bad effects. Well, this is bullshit. All I ever want to eat is pizza, which is basically a nuclear bomb of glycemic loads, and the more of it I eat, the fatter I get.

■ I should eat 39 to 44 grams of fiber a day. That's just good sense for good pooping. The FDA, for example, suggests

25 grams of fiber a day. The average American, though, only eats 16 grams a day.

- I can tolerate lactose. This is true—I've never experienced problems with dairy products.

- I am not at risk of overeating later if I skip a meal. This I've noticed to be the case whenever I do intermittent fasting. I just eat a regular meal when the time comes.

- I should eat protein from all kinds of sources, not particular ones, and I should spread it out evenly throughout the day. Apparently, some folks' genes say they should focus on getting their protein from certain sources for better absorption, or eating it at different parts of the day. Not me! But this is also pretty good common advice.

- I don't have sensitivity to most fats or salts. I honestly have no clue what this means, but it has something to do with my muscles.

- I could benefit from protein powder. Again, pretty standard.

- I should eat whole-grain food, but I don't need to actively push it into my diet. Again, a duh.

Nothing in here was mind-blowing. Most of this was standard advice. It was interesting to read that my genes said that I should be good with dairy products and I was good with skipping meals. I hadn't realized either thing about myself. Thanks, genes!

My genes and exercise

Finally, there was a big section on my workouts and, more important, what *kind* of workouts I should be doing.

- I should take a medium rest between sets. This is exactly what I do already. Thanks, science!

- I should perform exercises at a fast tempo. Already what I do.

- For resistance (i.e., strength) training, I should either do a low or a high number of sets. The most success I've seen, both in sticking to it as well as changing my body, has come when I've done this. I don't know if that's because most exercise routines I've encountered push for this kind of frequency or just because it worked for me, but still. Interesting to read. (Also: *This is how almost every popular weight lifting program works*—either low reps for strength or high reps for hypertrophy, or building muscle.)

- I'm likely to have an equal distribution of slow- and fast-twitch muscle fibers. Slow-twitch muscles help enable endurance exercises, such as distance training. Fast-twitch muscles are geared toward powerful movements, like sprinting or quickly lifting heavy weights. I'm someone who can run long distances and lift heavy weights, but do neither of them super great, so it makes sense that my muscle profile would match this.

- I have a medium recovery rate, so I shouldn't push past four strength sessions a week. Whenever I've done more than that, it's completely tanked me. So this rings true for me.

This section was by far the most spot-on of everything I'd read. It also made me wonder how much of this is just pretty standard for people or if I am truly some sort of outlier. I don't have access to anyone else's genes—and I wasn't paying to send in anyone else's DNA—so I don't know what it would say about other people.

But if the company encourages folks to eat more nutritious foods, exercise more, and get other lifestyle habits that lead to healthier lives, then I think it's not such a waste of money.

GENEALOGY DATABASES ARE HELPING SOLVE MURDERS

By the end of 2018, fifteen murder and sexual assault cases were solved because of a single genealogy website.[7] The main reason is that the site, GEDmatch, allows anyone to upload data.

So what did investigators do?

They took the data of suspects and uploaded it. Then they were able to find biological relatives or, in some cases, construct potential family trees.

This will probably start happening more and more, leading to more people being caught, but also perhaps leading to more false positives, too, I would assume.

And with data security becoming more and more of an issue as we use a wider array of online sites, the potential for our DNA to be used—or misused—in these instances will keep increasing.

In the future, I hope insurance companies and employers don't start to charge different rates based on what they find in our genes. *Gattaca* was a fun movie and all, but I'd rather it not become our lives.

As one point of hope, in 2019, GEDmatch did change its terms of service to require users to explicitly opt in for their DNA profiles to be included in law enforcement searches.[8]

SLEEP IS ACTUALLY IMPORTANT (SURPRISE!)

Your body needs sleep. (Duh.) There's a reason your body wants to sleep all the time. During meetings with your boss. During long car rides. During movies starring Gerard Butler as the romantic lead. All the time.

Your body needs to do this because it needs to fix all the crap you threw at it during your day. The mere act of living beats up your body, even if you're not exercising or doing anything strenuous.

Those eight hours are the equivalent of an elongated pit stop at a racetrack. Your tires need to be rotated, you need more gas, your alignment needs fixing. Without it, you'll get out of whack. And then you won't win the big NASCAR race! (I don't know enough about this sport to make a proper analogy, and I refuse to look it up. Some journalist I am.)

Studies show that if you sleep less or sleep poorly, you're more likely to gain weight and have trouble losing it. The more stressed you are, also, the worse you sleep.

Part of this, scientists think, is because when you sleep, you release growth hormones, which help with your metabolism. Sleep also affects your levels of cortisol, a hormone that can come from stress but also is related to your metabolism. If your sleep gets disturbed, that growth hormone may not get released at all or in the right amount you need, which messes with your metabolism and energy levels.

Other hormones could be affected, particularly the ones that help regulate your appetite and feeling of fullness. Isn't that great? Not only do you feel like crap after not sleeping enough, but now you're also going to be hungry. It's like your body is actively fighting against you.

One study showed that participants who got between five and six hours of sleep saw more weight gain than those who got seven to eight hours of sleep. And people who slept more than that also tended to have a higher body mass index. So *more* sleep isn't necessarily good for you, either—seven to eight hours is the sweet spot.

Know what else? Studies show that people who sleep too little are more likely to eat more food, abandon their other weight loss and exercise habits, and have a harder time losing fat mass.[9] Basically, getting a high-quality night of sleep is important on so many levels to your health efforts that it should be a big priority for you, along with eating healthy food.

There are a few other factors. Many people who are overweight also have sleep apnea, which is a condition where your breathing repeatedly stops and starts, or as I like to call it, the night chokes. This makes you sleep much worse and wake up tired and less energized than after a normal night's sleep. On top of that, studies show sleep apnea can also decrease testosterone in men, which also can lead to weight gain.[10]

At one point in my life, I had gained so much weight I developed sleep apnea. I had gotten so fat my body was like, "Let's kill him." I went to a doctor, who told me I could either use a Darth Vader–esque mask to sleep every night, or, he nonchalantly said, I could lose seventy pounds. I used the mask for a long time, but *also* lost the weight. My sleep apnea is much more under control, but I wouldn't have known about it if I hadn't seen a doctor.

All these things added together prove that having a great night's sleep is so important. Which means you should probably work harder at sleeping better. Here are some ways to do that:

1. **Do a sleep study.** Find out if you have any issues related to sleep. Sometimes they can be hormonal. Maybe you have sleep apnea. If your partner tells you that you snore a lot, or you stop breathing while you're sleeping (which was my case), or you've ever had one of those things where you wake up suddenly because you *snored yourself awake*, go see a sleep doctor to get tested for sleep apnea. Regardless, if your sleep sucks and the other things on this list don't help, seek the advice of a medical professional.

2. **Keep your bedroom cold.** We sleep better when the temperature is low, so lower the thermostat.

3. **Keep your bedroom dark.** Light messes up your circadian rhythm, which gives you a bad night's sleep. Wearing a sleep mask can help. (I wear one sometimes.) And light from screens, like from your phone or tablet, doesn't help, either.

4. **Have a regular bedtime.** I have an alarm on my phone that tells me when it's time to head toward bed. I do all my pre-sleep activities, such as brushing my teeth and changing out of my clothes, and then I go to bed.

5. **Use your bed only for sleeping.** (And sex.) You want to get your brain into the habit of knowing that when you start toward your bed, it's sleep time. If you watch television or play with your phone or read, it's training your brain to stay awake in bed. (Guess who has a television in his bedroom? Me. I am a hypocrite.) If you read in bed and find it easy to fall asleep, that's fine. But if not, then you should read elsewhere, preferably in another room.

6. **If you can't sleep, get up and do something in another room.** Go read a book, watch some television, listen to a podcast, work on that book your editor expects in June. Once you get tired, head back to bed.

Sleeping is one of the most important parts of weight-loss success and general health and fitness. Even if you're exercising and eating healthy, if your sleep is crap, your body won't be able to set your hormones right, digest food as well, and fix all the damage you've done to it. So get thee to bed!

GETTING MY 'ROID ON?

It's impossible to write a book about health and fitness without mentioning the s-word: "squats."

No, no, I kid. (But squats are also important, especially if you don't want to suffer from "tiny buttitis" like me.) It's time to talk about steroids.

In case you don't know what steroids are, they are synthetic hormones designed to treat medical ailments by pumping up your body's level of testosterone, a sex hormone that does all sorts of things.

That's their *intended* use. People take steroids for ailments such as lupus, gout, asthma, rheumatoid arthritis, and, shocker, *low testosterone.*

To put it bluntly, steroids can and do save lives.

They can also help someone get stronger, and with that, gain more muscle mass or recover faster from exercise. (This is one reason why conditioning-based athletes tend to get caught using them—it's easier to ride a bike in the mountains of France if you've got a hormonal boost.)

Like many things in life, steroids can also be abused and hurt you. And if you're taking them without a prescription, it's against the law.

But here's the dirty secret the fitness world doesn't like to publicize: Lots of folks you see on covers of fitness magazines with huge muscles use steroids. Many professional athletes use them. As do many actors and others whose livelihoods depend on how they look. Hell, I even know some guys who took steroids while they played football in small-town Nebraska.

Whenever I tell someone that I lift weights, steroids almost always come up. "Oh," they'll start to say, "I could get big muscles, too. All I have to do is take steroids. Super easy!"

No, it's actually not. You know those people who *do* take steroids? They still have to work out. They still have to push their bodies further than the average person does. Steroids allow people to bounce back from lifting weights faster, which allows them to continue to lift more, get stronger faster, and build muscle at a faster pace than someone not on the drugs.

I'm not here to make a moral judgment. I'm just saying—it's an option, and many take steroids. Because so many take steroids, it's warped our minds around beauty standards and what's possible naturally, especially for men. When you see a guy with gigantic arms and a huge, rippling chest, you think, "Gosh, if I just watch my diet and exercise properly, I could look like that, too!"

Maybe not. Because there's a chance that person's been using medical-grade enhancements to help him achieve that look, the kind you maybe don't legally have access to.

But before it sounds like I'm attacking those who use steroids, note that I'm not.

Because I almost became one of those people. For science!

Andy almost does steroids (for science)

When I started the research for this book, I had my blood analyzed. My doctor noticed my testosterone levels were kind of low, so he thought maybe it was an anomaly and had me come in and do another test. My testosterone was even lower the second time.

We're talking low. The median amount of testosterone for someone my age is 597, according to a 1996 study. I was at 194. That's low even for a seventy-five-year-old man.

On top of that, I was tired all the time, I was more irritable than usual, I had recently gained thirty pounds (again, *for science*), and I had a hard time focusing and completing things. All of which are signs of low testosterone in men.

My doctor immediately scheduled me for further tests with a few different specialists. Long story short, they concluded that nothing was physiologically wrong with me, and they were prepared to give me testosterone-enhancement therapy, which is a fancier way of saying, "We're going to give you a needle so you can shoot steroids into your butt."

One specialist asked me if my girlfriend at the time was a nurse, because then it would be easier for me to get a butt injection. I don't know if he asked all his patients if their significant others were medical professionals, but he asked me without a hint of sarcasm. He also gave me a grave look and asked if I was planning on marrying her, which I hadn't even thought about, let alone felt like discussing with a man who looked like he was delivering to me the worst news ever.

The doctor asked because steroids can make you infertile, and if I was planning on ever wanting children with my girlfriend, then he suggested she and I have a sit-down talk about it. (Narrator: They did not.)

I talked with a few of my weight-lifting friends before deciding. They were jealous: Steroids do wonders, they said. "Not that I would know or anything," they all immediately added, with a wink-wink. I'd be seeing sick gains in no time. "And it's legal!" they all told me, as if I had somehow won the steroid lottery.

After having made this decision, and deciding I would be okay with becoming sterile, I got a phone call from one of the specialists. They had me do one more set of blood work after all their other prodding and poking. Turns out, that blood work showed my testosterone increased up to around 350, which is a little low but well within a healthy range for someone my age.

I would not need testosterone replacement therapy after all. It was weird—I was kinda bummed. The world of steroid users was this thing I had heard so much about and is something we all probably see every day of our lives when we look at anyone with muscles in an advertisement. And I had a chance to legally do it! Under medical supervision! For science!

Instead, I would just use regular diet and exercise. Which is totally fine for me. And for you.

STEROID FUN FACTS

The main type of steroids used for fitness-related reasons are anabolic steroids, which are synthetic hormones that basically resemble testosterone, the male sex hormone. Testosterone promotes the growth of muscle, among many other things. Steroids can increase your strength, muscle size, and red blood cell production and can make you recover from exercise faster.

Many folks cycle on and off anabolic steroids, usually as an attempt to limit the negative side effects, which can include kidney problems, liver damage, an enlarged heart, and other cardiovascular issues.

In men, abusing steroids can lead to a decreased sperm count, a decrease in testicle size, baldness, an increased risk of prostate cancer, and the development of breasts. In women, they can cause the growth of facial hair, changes in menstrual cycles, and male-patterned baldness.

Do lots of people use steroids? Yes. Are many able to use them without any huge side effects? Yes. I won't judge someone for using steroids with a doctor's help. But the amounts used by some bodybuilders and others can be quite detrimental to one's health. It's not a miracle cure—and if you don't have a prescription, it's also illegal.

A last note about steroids: Many people use them in an attempt to speed up their metabolism. The science makes some sense. The more muscles you have, the more calories you can potentially burn at rest. But the truth is, you've got a lot of other ways to influence your metabolism.

YOUR METABOLISM PROBABLY ISN'T WHAT YOU THINK

You don't have a "slow" metabolism. Or a "fast" one. Others don't have them, either. You just have your metabolism, and it works however it's going to work.

Unless you have a very rare disease confirmed by a doctor, your metabolism is fine.

You are not overweight, or skinny, or anything because of your metabolism. It's an excuse I used to tell myself and others: *"My metabolism is pretty slow, and that's why I pack on weight so easily."* It's one excuse many of us like to tell about ourselves. Maybe even a doctor told you your metabolism was fast or slow, to which I would respond, uh, how would they know unless they did a specific test?

It's a reason we sometimes give to explain why people we know are skinnier than us. They're just *lucky*—their genes make them burn more calories than we do!

The reality is, we all don't have *that* much difference in our metabolism in the grand scheme of things. (Yes, we do have variations between our sexes, and because of things like height, muscle mass, and how much you exercise. But otherwise, we're all relatively similar.) Unless you've got a major medical problem, your body burns through fuel just like everyone else's, within maybe 100 calories a day.

Do 100 calories in either direction a day add up? Sure, they can. Over a period of a few months, that can be about a pound of weight in either direction.

Can you change your diet or increase your exercise to make that 100 calories not matter? You're darn right, you can.

You can burn 100 calories by running one mile or walking two. Or by not eating half a candy bar. Or by not drinking a soda.

Voilà—you've fixed that slow metabolism of yours.

Can you make your metabolism work differently? Kinda sorta. Your body will burn more calories in the hours after you do strength training than it would if you were just resting normally. And if you're a long-distance runner, that sort of training can make your body reconfigure *how* it metabolizes energy from your body.

And if you go into a hard-core calorie deficiency, you can slow down your metabolism during that diet. Some of this is because you actually have less body mass that needs to consume energy. And some of it could be because your body's slowing down your metabolism a little—but this doesn't mean it's ruined forever.

This is why some folks do what's called a "refeed" week, where, after a regular 500-fewer-calories-a-day restrictive diet, they then go back to their normal baseline. It's meant to tell your body, "Don't worry, I'm doing okay in the food world."

Also, remember in the last chapter we talked about how not all calories are equal? Depending on the kind of calories you consume—and how you prepare and eat them—you may be absorbing more or less of the calories than you think.

Regardless, you're more or less stuck with the metabolism you've got. You can make your body work a bit more efficiently with lots of exercise, but otherwise, it's going to do whatever it's going to do.

Don't think of it as bad. Just think of it as the mechanism that's keeping you alive!

My metabolism and me

I did a more advanced test to look at my metabolism, where I sat in a room and breathed into a tube that calculated how many calories

I use at rest. (You can do this, too, if you've got a few bucks.) According to the test, if I laid in bed all day and did nothing, I would burn 2,707 calories. That's *without* any extra activity. If I add in moving around during the day, plus exercise, I'm looking at burning about 3,500 calories a day, just to stay at a consistent weight.

When I was younger, I regularly said I was bigger because my metabolism was slow. Did I have any proof of this? Of course not. I said it to give myself an excuse, and to probably make me feel like I wasn't in control of my body. But the test I took showed the opposite: My metabolism is almost a quarter faster than the average person's.

To quote Maury Povich to my younger self: *That's a lie!* As it turns out, that was just another excuse I told myself, backed up by nothing.

But it also showed me something: I had been eating around 2,000 to 2,500 calories most days. By the end of the day, I'd be super tired. Turns out I wasn't eating enough.

I *was* losing weight, sure. But I also had no energy, especially when I exercised. That meant I had to eat a little more than I had first thought, which made my energy go back to normal. And I became a much happier human being.

You don't necessarily always have to have a caloric deficit to make your body look better, just for the record. You can maintain your weight and, through strength training, lose fat and gain muscle. It *is* possible. It doesn't happen for everyone, though.

But over time, if you're actively getting stronger or getting better at cardio-based activities yet staying the same weight, I guarantee you that your body is making changes. It may take you a few months to notice a change (this is why you should take before and after photos when embarking on any health or fitness changes), but trust me, it'll change.

ANDY DOES STEROIDS, SORTA?

Okay, you know how a few pages ago I said that I decided not to use steroids? I changed my mind about a year later. Sorta.

Months after the tests, some of the symptoms I'd had with low testosterone hadn't gone away. And new, more fun *issues* had started to appear. (Me and Bob Dole have things in common. I'm excited for my mom to read this sentence, and then we can never talk about it.)

My testosterone tests still showed my range as being well below average for my age. So instead of going back through the rigmarole of a big downtown Chicago medical center and a host of doctors who seemed more interested in what they could charge my insurance than in fixing me, I went somewhere else.

The internet.

I learned a lot more about hypogonadism, which is a fancy term for men who suffer from low testosterone. I also found it's becoming a bigger problem among men.

We have less testosterone than we used to! Studies continue to show declining testosterone levels in men and women today, compared with those of similar-aged people in the past. And doctors aren't really sure why.

One study showed that, starting in the 1980s, average levels for men's testosterone dropped about 1 percent per year. That means in 2004, a sixty-year-old man had testosterone levels 17 percent lower than a man who was that age in 1987.[11]

A study of Danish men showed the same—double-digit declines in testosterone among men born in the 1960s, compared with those born in the 1920s.[12]

Some explanations have been theorized: an increase in pesticide use that contaminated the foods we eat; more unhealthy lifestyles and obese people; fewer people working physically difficult jobs, which would make us more fit and produce more testosterone.

Whatever the reason, it's happening. And I'm proof! (Hooray!)

I found a lot of writing about testosterone-replacement therapy online, and almost everyone said that you don't treat what your charts say—like in my case, when my testosterone rates went into the mid-300s, it was "acceptable" but on the low side—but instead you treat the symptoms: my mood swings, my body-fat gain, my general fatigue. I found a doctor who specialized in these issues and made an appointment.

He said the same thing. Treat the symptoms. He was the first medical professional I felt actually listened to me.

He told me that I was doing the right things—eating relatively healthy, lifting weights, running, getting as much sleep as possible. He had me do some blood work, and after the results came in, we had another chat.

My testosterone was seriously low. And the other hormones he tested for, such as estrogen, were in the right range.

After an examination, where he applauded me on being tall (but still suggested I lose twenty pounds), he said I was incredibly healthy. And because I had done previous head scans and other work, and because of my blood work results, he didn't think anything was terribly wrong with me.

"For some reason," he told me, "your brain is telling your body not to produce testosterone."

To put it bluntly, my balls weren't working. He said perhaps there was some head trauma I'd had and forgotten about, but otherwise, he sort of threw his hands up in the air and said, "These things happen."

Instead of prescribing me testosterone, he was instead going to give me something called human chorionic gonadotropin, or HCG. This hormone can kick-start testosterone production in men.

Basically, it can get my boys to start doing their job.

It's a hormone I inject three times a week, along with taking a pill (Clomid) that is supposed to help, too.

Fun fact: HCG comes from the urine of pregnant women! And then I inject that into my body! ~*~*~science~*~*~

The reason he wanted me to do this, he said, was because of my age. Sometimes when you start testosterone therapy, you completely stop producing testosterone and, along with that, sperm. And then sometimes you can't start either back up.

So if I ever want to have kids, this would be the safer route. He also wanted me to get tested at a fertility clinic to see how my sperm production was doing, just to get a baseline for that.

So for three months, I'd try HCG. And if that didn't work, he'd put me on steroids. The real deal.

Injecting myself

Initially, it felt weird to inject myself with HCG and take Clomid three times a week. Even though a doctor was involved, and I did the research, I still felt like I was doing something illicit.

They're not *steroids* per se but sorta a precursor to my using them. It is a hormone. I've been doing something a bit unnatural to my body so I can see results similar to what I'd get if I *were* using steroids.

The first thing I noticed were the dreams. I've never been one to remember my dreams, at least in recent years, but that first week—good grief. I remembered *everything*. It was like I was dreaming more than I ever had in my life.

I mentioned it to a friend, and he was the first person to be like, "Maybe you're sleeping better?" I didn't even connect the fact that I was injecting myself with hormones with changes in my sleep patterns.

I wear a fitness watch to bed because I am cool, so I was able to check how much my sleep had changed. My watch tracks light sleep and deep sleep. The deep stuff is what you want a good deal of—

that's where the real work takes place in fixing your body and regu-
lating everything.

In the weeks leading up to my injections, I was getting one and a
half to two hours of deep sleep in an eight-hour night. I thought that
was pretty good.

But after two weeks of injections, it was more in the three-and-a-
half- to four-hour range. I was almost doubling the amount of deep
sleep I got every night.

Shocker: I woke up feeling more refreshed than I had in *years*. I
had more energy. A normal workout that would leave me exhausted
by the end? Now I felt not too shabby. I felt like I had a little extra in
the tank in case I needed it.

My moods improved. I felt more chipper. Could this be because
my testosterone levels were back to normal? Probably not—the doctor said it usually takes a month before you notice anything.

But could this be related to better sleep? Maybe!

Six months on HCG

Because the book-authoring process takes quite a while, I've had six
more months of taking HCG and Clomid. And here's what I've got
to show for it:

- Lost sixteen pounds
- Increased my testosterone rate, which has remained stable
  (still not amazing, but better than the rate of most eighty-
  year-old men)
- Continued to sleep much better
- Have much-less-erratic moods
- Continued to lift heavy weights and get stronger
- Continued to run long distances at a decent speed (9:30 a
  mile for a 10K)

My doc said one of the reasons I've been able to lose the weight is that my increased testosterone has helped with my moods, which pushed me toward making healthier decisions. And having more testosterone helps you keep off the fat. This is why lots of folks who are struggling with lifestyle changes in regard to their diets choose HCG or testosterone-replacement therapy.

Now, there is something called the HCG diet. It requires you to take HCG and then consume a ridiculously low number of calories a day—500 to 800 calories. Then, miraculously, you lose weight. This sort of ultra-low-calorie diet is bad for many reasons, which I explain in the next chapter. But it's not the HCG that's helping you lose the weight; it's the lack of calories.

My doctor did tell me that I needed to cut my caloric intake while on HCG, but only because it would help the medication be more effective. So, in that sense, I was on an HCG-oriented diet. It's just not the one you may read about online.

It's still kind of awkward to inject myself regularly, but the test results show that my testosterone level has gone up by more than 100, and most of my symptoms have disappeared. Still, I'm looking at losing another fifteen pounds, as my doctor says that'll lead to the treatments working even better. Here's to hoping that by the time this book is released, I'll have the testosterone of a normal guy in his thirties. (And, of course, that I'll no longer need these injections because my body's working normally again.)

6

How to Know if Someone Is Vegan (and Other Diets, Explained)

DIETS DON'T WORK

In life, we all have events we have to look nice for. A wedding, a beach vacation, your high school reunion. And because of these events, people try all sorts of things to look their best. Rent Lamborghinis, ask an attractive friend to pose as a spouse—all sorts of classics.

But what people also do is try to lose a ton of weight in a short period of time. These are called crash diets, and they are bad.

Similar to how a plane crashing is not good, neither is crash dieting.

When you do a crash diet, you limit the number of calories you eat to an extreme degree. For some, it may mean going from 2,500 calories a day to 500. That's the equivalent of going from three healthy meals throughout your day to eating just three chocolate-chip cookies.

Doing this for an extended amount of time is bad for a whole slew of reasons.

Your body will freak out. If you don't eat enough food to keep your body satisfied, it starts to go into damage control, sending signals to you nonstop saying, "HEY, EAT FOOD! YOU ARE GOING TO DIE."

You'll lose hair and have bad skin. If your goal is to try to lose weight in a short period of time in order to look good for something, having your hair fall out and blotchy skin may not be what you're going for.

You'll lose lots of muscle. When your body is freaking out and trying to find something to devour, it'll eat not only the fat on your body but also the muscle. So you won't end up looking slimmer, necessarily, but rather as a smaller version of how you already look.

Your mood will go haywire. You know the concept of being hangry, or hungry and angry, where your mood gets all out of whack and you act like a jerk and are super mean to loved ones? Cool, now imagine that times ten. And it's every moment of your life for a month. See? Not good.

Your concentration will go poof. Know what happens when you go on an extreme diet? Your brain goes into overdrive thinking you're going to die, and your thoughts revolve around eating. You constantly crave food.

Your sleep will be crap. If you have hunger pangs constantly, and your mind won't stop thinking about food, how well do you think you'll sleep? Not well, that's how!

It may not work. If you already are having issues with impulse control when it comes to food, what makes you think that suddenly deciding you're going to eat far less will help? It may not. We're not great at impulse control. It's one reason why many of us weigh more than we'd like. And we're being constantly bombarded with things to attack that lack of control, to force us to make purchases we don't want and eat things we shouldn't. While on a crash diet, you'll be more likely to end up saying, "To heck with this!" and going back to your old ways.

Even if it does work, you'll probably gain back the weight. Studies have shown that when people lose a ton of weight in a drastically short period of time, they may hit their goals, yes, but within months they not only gain the weight back but also put even *more* weight back on.

Remember when we talked about those evil hormones that deal with your appetite? They can get out of whack and freak out because you lost so much weight at such a fast pace. Your body tells you, "Let's prevent this from happening in the future. So you should pack on some more pounds to protect yourself!"

Your body doesn't know what you're trying to do. It can only react to outside stimuli. And when you go on a sudden, huge diet, it thinks you're about to starve and does everything it can to prevent you from dying. Think back to what our ancestors dealt with: regular droughts, bad hunting seasons, famine galore. You've been genetically engineered to deal with occasional bouts of no food. Your body knows how to protect itself in times of crisis.

If you've got a big event coming up that you want to lose some weight for, you should instead plan months and months ahead. I've said it before, but aim to lose one pound a week by *slowly* changing your eating habits and adding some exercise. Any weight loss beyond that—unless you're severely obese—means you're setting yourself up for potential trouble.

On top of that, even if you're trying to look gorgeous for these one-off events, you know what? You are already great-looking. If someone doesn't like how you look, or if some former high school crush is going to be awful to you because you don't look the same way you did in high school, to hell with them. You are who you are. You don't need their approval anyway.

But you *should* definitely rent a Lamborghini.

Important note: If you choose to be vegan or vegetarian or whateverian because of your beliefs, that's great. Don't let anyone tell you that you *must* eat meat or animal byproducts. What you decide to consume is up to you.

A BRIEF HISTORY OF DIETING

The first blockbuster diet book was written in 1864 by a British funeral director named William Banting.[1] He was a short and obese man who had dealt with his weight all of his life. He tried everything to lose the weight. Nothing worked.

Then he went to a doctor and asked what to do. The doc made Banting write down his daily diet. As a prescription, the doctor handed him a sheet of paper, telling him to stop consuming potatoes, bread, sugar, beer, and milk.

And it worked. Banting lost a lot of weight and decided he had to share it with the world.

The resulting book, *Letter on Corpulence*, was translated into French and German and sold many copies in Europe and the United States. His name means "diet" in Swedish, and for a long time, the phrase "to bant" meant "to diet."

Basically, Banting invented the low-carb diet.

WORRYING ABOUT OUR WEIGHT

Part of the problem with dieting is that so much of the "blame" for our obesity is thrown onto the individual: It's a moral failing that you're overweight. You're stupid. You're bad. You're to blame.

I've felt this throughout my whole life. Repeatedly, when I was heavier, doctors would bring up my weight constantly.

One time, I went in because I had strep throat. (They did a test and everything!) The doctor was like, "Yup, you've got strep throat. Also, are you aware that you're obese?"

No, Doctor. I wasn't aware whatsoever. It never came up. Egad, you're blowing my mind right now. Please tell me more.

She then went on to say that if I just dieted and exercised I'd be in better shape. "Young, smart guy like you," she said, shaking her head, "you should know better."

Almost half of Americans are worried about their weight all or some of the time, according to a Gallup poll.[2] Of those Americans who consider themselves already overweight, two-thirds are more likely to worry about their weight than those who say their weight is "about right."

On top of that, the same poll showed a majority of Americans who view themselves as overweight said they were actively trying to lose weight. That means so many people are not only struggling with their weight, but they're actively trying to feel better about it.

The data isn't good, either. According to the *American Journal of Public Health*, an obese person's chance of achieving a "normal" weight is less than 1 percent.[3]

We've known this for a *long, long, long* time. Since the late 1950s, research has shown that two-thirds of people who lose weight on a diet gain back more than they lost.

Let me repeat that: The majority of people who try to lose weight through dieting not only fail, but they actually get heavier. And depending on the research you read, the chance of failure when you try to lose weight is potentially quite high. (The medical literature is somewhat sticky on an actual percent, because many argue that the diets are failing people, not people failing the diets, and some of the numbers are based on studies more than sixty years old.)

Being overweight does not mean you're unhealthy. While you may see positive health effects from losing weight, I don't want you to think that losing weight is the be-all, end-all of fitness.

Larger people can be healthier than skinnier people, for instance, when it comes to blood pressure, blood test results, and physical ability. So if your weight is on the high side, don't think you need to become super skinny to be healthy.

What you may need to do instead is change your eating habits. It's not a *diet*; it's instead just how you now eat.

It's not meant to be done for a short time. If you want to enact change, you gotta get into it for the long haul.

Exercise is also important, as I said in the previous section. What you can do with your body is, in my opinion, more important in the long run than how your body looks. But what you're able to do with your body also changes because of what you put into it.

I go into more specifics later in the book, but here's the basic facts of a healthier diet: Eat fewer sugary carbs, more fats, more protein, and fewer processed foods. Prepare more of your meals yourself. Drink more water.

That's a diet you can believe in.

Detox diet? More like detox bullshit

Do you have at least one working kidney? How about your liver— does it also work? Are you currently *not* hooked up to a dialysis machine?

If you answered yes to all these questions, guess what? Your body detoxes itself just fine! You don't have to eat cayenne peppers, go on a lime-juice fast, or do any other crazy nonsense diet in order to "cleanse" your body.

People peddle this nonsense all the time about how eating this particular thing or drinking these certain liquids will somehow help clean out all the unnatural things in your body. That's what your kidneys and liver are for, folks. If they weren't working properly, you would get sick.

And possibly turn yellow.

Oh, and die.

Your body works just fine to naturally cleanse itself of so-called impurities. It's already done "naturally." Nobody has some sort of magic cleansing diet or liquid to cure what ails you. If someone is feeding you that kind of goop, they don't know how the body works. They're also hoping you don't either, so they can profit off you.

On top of that, you probably shouldn't listen to their advice about anything else related to your body. Because it sounds like they're *maybe* more interested in selling you the equivalent of cayenne pepper–flavored snake oil than something that actually helps you.

"But, Andy," you're telling me, "I totally feel different after doing it!" You probably do! If you fast and don't consume anything other than spicy water, I bet that will make your body feel a bit different. Doesn't mean you've somehow been cleansed of toxins.

"But, Andy," you're still telling me, "when I was on my cleanse I lost *five pounds*! In only a week!" I bet you did lose five pounds! Because you haven't eaten any real food. Or had much salt in your diet. And you're probably dehydrated. You've just lost a lot of water weight but no real weight. (Plus, your bowels are empty, too, which means you have less poop weight, which, trust me, is a thing.)

Not to mention, as I've said many times before, losing five pounds in a week isn't healthy. As soon as you get some non-cleansing food in your body, you'll "gain" back that weight you never really lost.

"But, Andy," you are now yelling at me from what I assume is a fast car, like a '68 Mustang, "I know someone else who said this really helped them and was awesome!" That's great. I'm glad for this stranger you allegedly know. I do think "cleanses" and things like that have a nice placebo effect and could possibly help push you to make better choices about your health.

If that's why you're doing it, awesome! If you're doing it because you think your body needs regular cleansing, that's not awesome.

You'll be fine if you just eat normally. Save the deep cleanses for your bathtub.

Intermittent fasting

In the past few years, a new kind of diet method has been getting lots of attention. It's called "intermittent fasting," and it's something I've done off and on. It's a pretty simple concept: Limit the times when you eat food.

Here's an example: Instead of having your regular 8:00 a.m. breakfast, noon lunch, and 7:00 p.m. dinner, you decide, "I will eat only from noon until 8 p.m." You have an eight-hour window when you'll have meals, and sixteen hours when you don't eat.

It's just a method of cycling between periods where you eat and periods where you fast. It's not about dieting and changing what and how much you eat, so much as it is about changing *when you eat*.

I know bodybuilders who swear by it, and people who've lost a ton of weight who also say it's great. Not to mention, many doctors also suggest it as a great weight-loss method, and many studies have been done to show its positive effects.[4]

A few types of intermittent fasting have become popular lately:

The eight-hour method

This is the one I described above, in which you give yourself an eight-hour window to eat food each day. It more or less involves skipping breakfast and then having lunch, a snack, and then dinner. Then you're done with your daily food intake.

We're all told that breakfast is the most important meal of the day, which is a slogan invented by people who sell breakfast food. The problem is, most people who skip breakfast usually have bad eating habits to begin with. Or for breakfast they eat carb-heavy cereal or some other high-calorie junk, such as a bagel (I know, they're delicious).

By following this form of intermittent fasting, you're attempting to rein in some of your bad habits by creating new good ones.

If you usually eat a 600-calorie breakfast, and now you no longer have those calories, you've more than hit enough of a deficit to lose a pound a week. Just make sure that the rest of your meals aren't exponentially larger. And as I've suggested previously, make sure you're eating a good amount of protein and fats so you stay satiated and have the energy you need.

If this seems too difficult, try easing into it. Instead of fasting for an eight-hour window, maybe try ten at first.

The twenty-four-hour fast

In this method, for one or two days a week you don't eat from dinner one day until dinner the next. Or from lunch to lunch. Or breakfast to breakfast.

It sucks.

I hate it.

I've tried it, and I don't think it's a good method. I'm including it in this list because I've known others who have used it in the past and have *somehow* been able to do it.

It's not the best idea, especially if you already have problems with eating, because you'll instantly want to binge the next time you get a chance to eat. It defeats the whole purpose of fasting.

Not to mention, for many of us, unless fasting has become something we've gotten accustomed to through religious reasons, it's hard to break that cycle of having regular meals. The one week I tried to do this I just about went insane, as everything in my body told me I should run down the street and have a candy bar.

On top of this, if you exercise at all, you'll have no energy because your body's reserves will most likely be completely depleted. It's Suck City (Population: You).

Two hell-days fast

This method has you eat only 500 to 600 calories for two days a week, as long as they're not consecutive. You could have a Tuesday and a Thursday where you eat only 600 calories, and then the other days you eat normally.

This intermittent fasting method is normally known as the 5:2 diet, but let's give it its real name: Ugggggghhhhhhhhhh. (I'm going to patent that.) I also tried this diet, and even though I was able to do it, it was damn hard. You dread those two days, because you know you basically get *one* meal a day. And you better make it high in protein and fats or else you'll start to get hunger cravings immediately.

And again, if you exercise, it's going to suck because your body will be completely depleted, and you'll just want to sit on your couch watching TV shows you've already watched ten times on Netflix over and over and over.

Finally, if you give in and have a lot of carbs with that one meal, as I did one time when I gave in to a candy bar, you will become carb crazy and want to eat *every* cracker and piece of bread within a five-mile radius. Nobody wants that, unless you're a bread or cracker farmer.

■ ■ ■

Based on my highly scientific research (it was not highly scientific), I would suggest the eight-hour method of fasting for most people, especially if you're new to the whole thing. Some say this method also mimics our evolutionary needs, because only during the last sixty years has obtaining so much food become so much easier.

An important note for women: Intermittent fasting *can* affect your hormones and your menstrual cycle, which can make it counterproductive to weight loss. Not everyone is affected, but intermittent fasting isn't always as effective for women as it is for men.

Instead of plunging straight into an eight-hour fasting method every day, women who've never tried intermittent fasting should fast for two or three nonconsecutive days a week—a Monday, Wednesday, and Friday, for instance. If you notice any major changes in your body, mood, stress level, or appetite, then you should stop and talk to your doctor before trying again.

Here are some more reasons why you should try intermittent fasting, regardless of your gender, if other methods to help you get your eating on track have failed:

1. **It limits calories.** If you're having fewer meals during the day, you're more likely to eat fewer calories overall. Now, if you decide to make your meals twice as large as they previously were, that won't help. But if you decide to just skip breakfast and then eat your regular lunch and dinner, you're no longer consuming those breakfast calories.

2. **It may boost your metabolism.** Studies have shown your energy expenditure, or the number of calories your body burns at rest, can increase when you're depriving yourself of calories for longer periods.[5] Even though you *do* eventually eat, and you may even eat a regular number of calories, as on the previous day, your body can burn more of them off without your doing anything extra.

3. **Your insulin sensitivity can improve.** Your insulin levels won't go up and down as much, meaning you won't get those serious hunger pangs because of an insulin crash—like the feeling you get after eating a Twinkie (don't judge me) and an hour later you're barely able to stay awake at your desk. Intermittent fasting can also drop your levels of insulin, which makes it easier for your body to reach stored fat as an energy source.

4. **It can be easier than traditional diets.** Reducing the time during which you consume food during the day means less time that you have to concern yourself with following all the specific rules of traditional diets. That means fasting could be easier for you to follow than other diets that might have failed in the past.

5. **It can help you lose belly fat.** Even though I think this is tied more to the overall caloric restriction, one study showed that people who intermittently fasted saw a reduction in their waistline.[6] Having less belly fat is overall healthier for you.

6. **It has other health benefits.** Studies have shown that intermittent fasting can help you in a myriad of other ways, including increased brain health (in tests using mice,)[7] reduced inflammation,[8] and lower heart-disease risk factors.[9]

7. **It may help you live longer.** Other than the standard health benefits of losing weight, some studies show it could potentially extend your lifespan. One study showed that male mice were able to live, on average, 83 percent longer when they fasted every other day, compared with mice that ate daily.[10] (This is especially good news for you, dear reader, if you happen to be a literate mouse.)

If you've been having trouble counting calories or using other methods to reduce the amount of food you regularly ingest, try intermittent fasting. This method may work better for you.

Reducing the amount of time when you're eating means you're more likely to eat less. It's an easy way to help you combat the potential for getting the munchies and has some added benefits that can help you toward your goal of being a healthier you.

It's another sneaky way to trick yourself into eating fewer calories.

Ketosis and peeing on strips (for science)

Read enough about weight loss and fitness and you'll hear of a cure-all called the ketogenic diet. Folks swear by it, saying that it helped them lose lots of weight.

It works like this: Your body likes to use blood sugar as its main source of energy, which we often get from carbohydrates. But if you don't have any of that blood sugar floating around—because you aren't eating a lot of carbs, essentially—then your body switches to breaking down your fat cells into something called ketone bodies, in a process called ketosis.

Until you start eating carbs again, your body will continue to break down those fat cells and produce ketones. It usually happens for folks who eat between 20 and 50 grams of carbohydrates a day.[11]

For reference, two slices of white bread contain about 30 grams of carbs. Because ketosis is a pretty low-, low-, low-carb diet, people on it end up eating foods high in protein and fats; it usually also requires you to cut out most processed foods.

(This is how a lot of bodybuilders eat, by the way: low-carb, high-protein, and high-fat foods, without any, or very few, processed foods.)

Keto is nothing new. Doctors have been using it for a century to treat patients with drug-resistant forms of epilepsy. It started to become popular in the 1970s after Dr. Robert Atkins pushed it as part of his low-carb diet plan.

I tried the keto diet years ago. It worked super well. You can discover if it's actually working only by peeing on test strips that tell you the number of ketones your body is producing. (That's a fun daily activity to explain to people.)

I lost about twenty pounds in a few months. It required me to eat healthier and make better choices, all of which worked out.

The problem?

Eating that few carbs for a long period of time was so mentally draining. It was like fighting an uphill battle every day.

That meant I eventually broke down and started eating carbohydrates again. First, I did it at a few cheat meals. Then on cheat days. Then cheat weeks. Then I "forgot" to test my pee, and soon I was no longer doing the keto diet.

Sound familiar to any diet you've tried?

A keto diet can work, sure, but I think it should be paired with something else *after* you've seen the initial weight loss. Get to a healthier weight and then find food options that make sense so that you can maintain the weight you're at.

The goal shouldn't be to constantly attempt to lose weight. Get to a manageable weight while doing ketosis or any diet. I know it's a lot harder than it sounds, as I struggle with my weight on a regular basis.

Also, it means you'll be peeing way less on test sticks, which I always consider a plus.

Studies have shown the keto diet is safe for long- and short-term use.[12] In tests, it's been shown to significantly reduce the weight and body mass index of obese patients. Their blood work results also became substantially better, and the diet didn't lead to any significant side effects.

Is it because this diet melts off fat? Sort of. But the more important thing, I believe, is that this kind of diet pushes you to eat fewer calories.

You're losing weight because it's burning your fat cells, sure, but also because a ketogenic diet forces you to stop eating a lot of crappy foods. Which, as in many other diets, means you eat fewer calories.

It's a method of tricking you into eating less without your *knowing* you're doing that. That's why these low-carb diets work. It's not just that your body is reacting to the food differently; it's that you're consuming less.

The paleo diet, straight outta modern times

One popular diet that works—and is loved by many ketogenic enthusiasts—is the paleo diet.

The thinking behind the paleo diet is that we should eat like our ancestors did ten thousand years ago. That means focusing on what hunters and gatherers ate.

So, a diet that includes lean meats, fish, vegetables, fruits, nuts, and seeds. Not on this list? Dairy products, legumes, and grains.

That's the diet. As with many of the other diets I've mentioned, it means you can't eat processed foods. It means your sugar intake will plummet.

Regardless of whether this is what people actually ate back then (and research says it probably wasn't), lots of folks live by it.

I tried it for one month. I lost twenty pounds.

Was this because I was also training for a half marathon and running a few dozen miles a week? Maybe!

Could it be because the month before I had eaten a lot because I was super stressed at work, and it was the holidays and cookies were everywhere, so I had probably an extra ten pounds of dessert and water weight that caused my starting weight to be skewed? Also maybe!

But the paleo diet limited my food intake, got me to eat healthier, and made my decisions about food a lot better. (And because of the low-carb, no-processed-food part, I probably went into ketosis. But I wasn't peeing on any strips to find out.)

The only hard part came when I would be out with friends or at parties. Someone would have a food tray out, or maybe cupcakes. I'd eye them and know I couldn't eat them. People would ask me what's up. One dude was like, "You're at a birthday party—*you need to be eating cake or it's weird.*"

So I got a piece of cake and I felt *so guilty* taking a bite of it. That's one thing this diet can do to you—or any diet can do to you: make you feel bad about your food decisions.

Don't fall into that trap. Just view this diet, or any diet, as more of a guideline. You should still be able to enjoy yourself and eat tasty things on occasion. (Moderation is everything, of course.)

If you're looking for a diet that's no frills and easy to do, try paleo. It doesn't make you better than other people. It won't turn you into a caveman. But it can get you started on some better habits. And maybe it can make you go ketogenic.

7

Exercise Is Important, but How Important, Really?

ANDY TRAINS FOR A HALF MARATHON

I was miles from my hotel when terror struck me. I was on an early-morning training run because I had stupidly told my editor that, for this book, I would train for and run a half marathon, just so I could write about it. And now I was in the middle of nowhere—also known as Lincoln, Nebraska—during a book tour for my previous book. And I had to go to the bathroom really, really bad.

I don't know if you've ever been in a Midwestern industrial corridor at 7:00 a.m. and really had to take the Browns to the Super Bowl, but let me tell you, it sucks.

Before I tell you how that story ended, and before I walk you through the idiocy of training for a half marathon, let's get a bit of science out of the way when it comes to endurance training. A 2007 study followed some postmenopausal women who were overweight or obese as they tried different methods of light cardio exercise.

The study found that just ten minutes a day of light walking for six months increased peak oxygen consumption, a measure of cardiovascular health, by 3.8 percent. Folks who almost doubled that time? They saw a 6.7 percent increase. Those who *didn't* do any exercise during that time? Their cardiovascular health dropped by 1.7 percent.[1]

But those who do tons and tons more? Diminishing returns.

Running more and more and more and more and more doesn't nec-essarily give you *that* big of a bump, according to that study.

Almost all my public education promoted running as the best way to get in shape. A lot of the fitness world focuses on it, too—cardio is this alleged cure-all. Not to mention, most fitness classes are usually cardio-based.

While I never did any cardio other than long walks in my initial attempts at getting in better shape, I thought it only fair that I try a bunch so I could write about it. To run a few dozen miles in other people's shoes, so to speak.

Running *does* burn calories. And because I'm a bigger guy, I burn more than someone who is smaller does. So that definitely could help me with my weight-loss goals. But just losing weight doesn't lead you to necessarily having the physique that's ideal by Western standards, if that's what you're going for. (And for me, yeah, I am.)

Yet time and time again, through high school and college, I heard that the only way I could get in better shape would be by running a lot. You know what's a good way to motivate yourself into running a lot? Get a book deal where you're contractually obligated to train for a half marathon.

My training plan basically had me running four days a week, slowly upping the miles during those sixteen weeks until I was able to complete a 13.1 mile run with no walking.

During my training, I decided to focus mostly on running. I didn't lift weights all that much—maybe once or twice a week. Whenever I did, I wasn't trying to break new records in terms of strength. It was maintenance mode, if that, on account of how dead tired I was after all my running. And, let's be honest, I let my eating habits slide a bit. In my mind, I told myself *because* I was running so much, I needed the energy, and I'd be burning it off anyway, right?

Wrong.

What tended to happen was the opposite. I'd overeat, going way over the number of calories I needed. I saw the scale creeping up and up. What'd I do then? Usually I stopped looking at the scale. When I regularly tracked my weight, I'd manage to keep myself in check and either stay around the same weight or slowly lose a pound or two a week.

Let's jump back to where I was in Lincoln. I was in town for a week, staying at a hotel next to the state penitentiary because I didn't look at a map before booking my lodgings. An old college friend who's a prison guard told me the spot I picked is where inmates usually immediately go when they're released to, uh, *reconnect* with their wives and girlfriends.

The perfect place to decide to go for a run.

I was about two miles away from my hotel when the stomach pain hit me. This was about four weeks into my marathon training. When you run in Chicago, if you've got to stop to take a break or find a restroom, odds are you're running in a neighborhood and can find a helpful coffee shop willing to take in a super-sweaty dude. But not in the industrial wasteland of south Lincoln.

Did I mention this was next to the state pen? That's where they used to electrocute people! (I know this because in college I got a tour of the prison and they showed us the room where Old Sparky lives. Yes, they actually called it that.)

I was on a random road when I saw a semi pulling into a nearby long building, which I assumed was where the state kept all its corn secrets. I followed the vehicle, running while simultaneously holding my gut, and a guy got out, whom I shall call Diesel on account of my never learning his name. I explained my predicament. Being the nice Midwestern man that he was, and noticing I was a super sweaty guy in running gear, Diesel let me follow him into the place and use the bathroom.

He kept close guard until I left the building. As I was leaving, he asked what I was doing.

"Training for a half marathon," I told him.

"That's dumb," he said, laughing as he shut the door behind me. Diesel was right.

This was one of the many signs that training for a half marathon was going to be a lot harder than I expected.

After I returned to Chicago, the training continued. The temperature rose, my runs got longer, and I started to learn the true meaning of pushing yourself. Many days I did not want to go for my six-mile "easy" run, but I did it. I realized the importance of drinking water after suffering from what I'm pretty sure was heat exhaustion, and I purchased myself a water-bag thingy to wear on my back, like I was a little kid going to school, except all my books were water and I drank them. (This metaphor is bad.)

I wore out my shoes a few times. I learned that if I didn't wear the right kind of socks, the run would become the worst thing ever, as blisters would swiftly appear. I also learned that a man's nipples are tender, and they don't appreciate my running without safety precautions (aka wearing nipple guards; nothing is cuter than having a bunch of nipple-based blood stains on the front of your running shirt in Manhattan following a run during a New York City work trip).

Overall, what I learned was this: Almost anyone can train for a long-distance race. But just because you do, you don't magically get in better shape. I lost some weight, but I didn't *look* any better, compared with how I looked in previous photos I had taken of myself. I was mostly always a little red, on account of my species of white person being unable to tan whatsoever. (My friend Tyler tried to take me tanning when we were seniors in high school. I was so sunburned I couldn't move without pain for about three days. Never again.)

I wasn't staying on track with my food, so I was mostly just treading water, in terms of my weight and how I looked in my progress photos, even if I was becoming more athletic, able to run longer and longer, somehow pushing myself on my long runs to go distances I never, ever thought possible. The longer I ran, the more my body hated me. The more my knees hurt. The more just a "short" run of five miles would cause my right knee to somehow give out.

And just one week before race day, my right knee started regularly hurting so bad I had to stop running altogether, for fear I would injure myself further. I had a week to rest before the big day.

Little did I know what hell awaited me on race day.

WEIGHT LIFTING, AND WHY YOU SHOULD DO IT

Before I regale you with a tale that took me through hell, I'd first like to walk you through a bit of heaven. Or rather, what I think is quite angelic. (And is probably how Saint Michael the Archangel got his well-defined pecs.)

All my research has pointed to one type of exercise that folks repeatedly say gets you the best results in the most efficient way possible: strength training.

Lifting weights.

More specifically, lifting weights with a barbell. Or as I call it, going to the iron church to pray to the lord of gains. (I do not call it that, but I thought adding to the religious imagery would help.)

That means using one of those long pieces of iron, putting weights on the sides, and then using your body plus gravity to move it. It can be scary, it can be hard, but the science shows it's one of the best ways for you to build and maintain muscle mass when combined with a good diet.

Note the most important words there: "a good diet."

If you continue to eat like trash, or at least don't curb *some* of your more trash-like eating, no matter how often you do cardio or lift weights, you won't see any improvement.

You can't out-fit a bad diet.

Not everyone wants to lift weights. I get it. But think of it this way: You know people who have physiques you envy? While they have their own bodies, their own genetics, their own past choices, how do you think the vast majority of them got to look the way they do?

Exercise that involved strength.

One example I'll cite is Alison Brie. She's an actress known for her roles on *Community* and *Mad Men,* and also for being just a delightful human being.

But when she wanted to take on the role of Ruth Wilder on the Netflix series *GLOW,* or *Gorgeous Ladies of Wrestling,* she stopped doing one thing that had been a regular part of her exercise routine.

Cardio.

She was in generally good shape, she told one magazine, but she wanted to be able to do all her own stunts.[2] That meant she needed some help, and to rethink her fitness plan.

Instead, while working with a trainer, Brie focused on one thing: getting as strong as possible.[3] That meant traditional barbell work, such as deadlifts, squat variations, and hip thrusts. It also meant pull-ups, push-ups, and other work focusing on her core.

The goal was to get as strong as she possibly could, her trainer, Jason Walsh, told *Self* magazine.

Now, while most of us don't need to prepare to portray a wrestler in the ring, the same sort of strength exercises Brie worked on are what many folks do in the gym to get stronger.

The stronger you are, the bigger your muscles get. The bigger your muscles get, the more visually appealing—in a traditional, Western sense—you generally are.

This goes for men and women. From a health perspective, more muscle means you burn more calories at rest. Not to mention, having less fat mass reduces your chances of having all sorts of diseases as well as heart attacks.

Stronger is better. And strength training gets you stronger.

Using just your body weight to train itself works, too. As do other forms of exercise, such as yoga and Pilates and anything else that requires you to *move* against a band or fight gravity.

But using a barbell—or dumbbells or machines—will get you more results in less time, and the studies show this.

That doesn't mean you can't do other things, though. The best exercise routine is the one you keep doing.

I would suggest following a barbell-based routine for a few months at some point in your life. You'll be surprised at how strong you are, and how strong you can get. It's been one of the most rewarding exercise styles I've ever done.

(For more on this, read a book such as Mark Rippetoe's *Starting Strength*, or check out one of the popular beginner barbell programs online. Just pick one and try it for a few months.)

"But I don't want to get bulky!"

Let's clear up some misconceptions about what happens when you lift weights.

When you lift a dumbbell a few times, your body does not suddenly go into a crazy state of shock, causing your entire DNA to change instantly, making muscles bulge and burst from all over your person.

Yet many folks say the same thing when you suggest they should lift weights to help them get healthier: "But I don't want to get bulky."

Many folks think that if you go to the gym you'll automatically end up looking like the Incredible Hulk. (Lou-Ferrigno era, not CGI-Marvel-action-film era.) The stereotype seems to be that everyone ends up with the same goal: to look like professional bodybuilders.

Now, there is nothing at all wrong with bodybuilding. In my pursuit of a healthier me, I've lifted the same way bodybuilders do. I've tried to eat like them as well. I've even attended bodybuilding competitions, just to learn more about the sport. (That story comes later in this chapter.)

But those people are aberrations, not the norm.

If you practice shooting baskets a few times a week, you wouldn't think you'd automatically get to the same level as LeBron James, would you? No, you'd have to practice a lot more, invent a time machine so you can start learning to dunk at age three, and you still wouldn't be as good as King James. Same thing with lifting weights—your body won't instantly turn into that of a bodybuilder overnight.

Bodybuilders are athletes. You can be an athlete, too, but they've got a big head start on you. Not to mention that many of them, uh, use other methods to reach their huge size. (And I'm not just talking about their already stellar genetics.)

On top of that, do you know what these people have to do to get that huge? They eat insane amounts of food—some eat more than five thousand calories a day, with giant meals every hour or two. They work out every day for hours. They also do tons of cardio. They usually sleep more than the average person because their bodies need a lot of rest to recover from all the damage they've done to them.

For many of these people, tending to their physiques is their full-time job. Not everyone has that time, nor should everyone be forced to act like that to seem "normal."

For many of us, lifting weights and eating a good diet causes us to end up with a slightly slimmer body, and maybe some more defined muscles. Maybe you finally get a noticeable booty when you've never had one previously. (Still not me. *Sigh.*) Maybe your face looks a bit skinnier. Or your shoulders appear broader.

But most people who go to the gym don't have to worry about hulking out and suddenly becoming huge and bulky.

Case in point: My mom, god bless her, is [AGE REDACTED

BY MOM LAW]. And when I suggested she lift some weights, her first response was, "I don't want to end up looking like Arnold Schwarzenegger."

Mom, I love you. But, c'mon.

You mean the guy who started lifting weights in his teens, admitted to using steroids, spent decades regularly competing in bodybuilding competitions, and centered his whole life on building muscles through diet and exercise? You don't want to end up looking like that?

For most of us, it's not going to happen. *And that's totally okay!* You don't *have* to look super muscular and buff like Arnold to be healthy. You can have body fat! You can have a little definition in your arms! That is all okay.

And for most of us, that's how we'll look after lots of exercise. I've been lifting weights regularly for three years, and I still have a bit of a gut. My arms look a little better than they used to, and my face is certainly slimmer. But still, I don't look like a muscle-bound freak.

You don't have to, either.

If you want to, that's also fine! Just know that it doesn't happen overnight, or by accident. It's years of work. Don't worry about getting bulky. Just be excited about getting healthy.

You can't "tone" anything

Speaking of which, our body is a big ol' complicated system, with different parts of it affecting how other parts work. But what it tries to do is spread the work out. Especially when it comes to where your fat cells live.

Men often retain their fat in their bellies. For women, it's in their hips. Thanks, genetics! There's not much you can do about it. What you *definitely* can't do is attempt to work out just a specific part of your body and make the fat go away in just that area.

This is a crap concept called "toning," or sometimes "spot reduction." You'll get some fitness guru who tells you that if you do lots of bicep curls, you'll lose fat on your arms. Or if you do a bunch of crunches, your belly will disappear. Or if you do lots of leg lifts, your butt size will decrease. (Who wants this?)

It's all a lie.

Other than in your genetically predisposed areas where fat concentrates, your fat is evenly spread out across the rest of your body. If you lose five pounds, you don't lose five pounds *only* in your left arm, or your right butt cheek, or your middle lower back. You lose it more or less evenly throughout your entire body, or at least proportionally, given your body's differently sized parts. (This is where your genes can sometimes be quite fickle, proving we are all, in fact, unique snowflakes.)

Think of it as a puddle of water evaporating. It usually starts out as a circle, and then it becomes a smaller and smaller circle, decreasing in time as more of it floats off into the atmosphere. That's what your body does when it comes to fat loss. You lose it throughout your entire body, regardless of *where* you work out.

Can you work out specific parts of your body and make those muscles bigger? You most definitely can! But for many of us, you first need to lose the fat that's on top of those muscles. Many people you envision as mega-ripped, or who have amazing arms and legs and whatever, actually just have lower body fat. They're just skinny, so their muscles pop.

At a higher body-fat percentage, you may actually have *bigger* muscles than they do, in terms of pure muscle size. But because you have more layers of fat on top, those muscles are harder to see.

Imagine a gigantic slab of marble. It's not a statue, is it? But if it gets chiseled away by a talented artist—poof!—it can be turned into something. That's what you're doing by lowering your overall body weight, revealing more of the statue inside you. (Hopefully pigeons don't poop on you.)

If you want to make a certain part of your body pop when you're overweight, there's only one scientifically proven method to do it: lose fat all over your body.

Fun fact: This chapter reminds me of one of my mom's favorite sayings: "Don't make up quotes and attribute them to me."

PROGRESSIVE OVERLOAD MAKES EXERCISE WORK

Remember homeostasis? Your body adapts. That includes adapting to the stressors you put on it.

Exercise works like this: You do something difficult, and your body adapts, helping you to make it less difficult the next time around. Then you make it harder, gradually increasing the difficulty every time you do the same exercise. This is called progressive overload.

With cardio, your body and cardiovascular system respond, working more effectively, helping you to run, row, swim, whatever, better the next time around. This is why when people train for runs, they usually have "pace" and "speed" days built in, to push themselves so their bodies will adapt to the harder runs.

With strength training, you break down muscle fibers by doing the movements. Then a few days later, as long as you've eaten and rested enough, you should be stronger. This is how someone can go from bench pressing 150 pounds to 300 pounds over a long period of time.

Progressive overload is the key to any and all exercise. If it's not built into whatever exercise plan you're following—whether it be cardio, strength training, or just going for walks—then you won't see any improvement in the area you're training.

Cardio classes

Cardio is big business and it's only getting bigger. If you walk around most major cities, you'll see new studios offering a variety of methods geared toward making you sweat your ass off, and promising that if you do what they say, you'll lose weight and get fit.

One of the reasons for this explosion is that it's easier to make more money by offering cardio than other forms of exercise. Let me give you an example from my youth.

I was in Jazzercise. Yeah, I know. I was *very* cool in elementary school. I was one of two boys and two dozen girls. And we had one instructor. Occasionally we would do our routines at malls, senior centers, and other places.

But think of the equipment we needed—nothing other than our clothes, perhaps some polyester dance outfits, and the roller rink we practiced at in my small town. A few dozen kids' parents paying a bunch of money for a class that requires only a single teacher.

The same applies to a lot of cardio-oriented classes. For many, you don't need much equipment or training, yet you can pack a ton of people into a single space, get them done in an hour or less, and then usher in the next group of people.

Selling some Soul

One of the big recent fitness crazes are spin classes, which is a fancier way of saying "sitting on a bicycle and sweating while pop songs from your middle school days are played and a peppy person says happy things at you while you pedal."

Lots of gyms offer spin classes, with whole areas cordoned off for them. They're usually the most packed classes, too. But one of the biggest players in the spin-class craze is SoulCycle.

The company was founded in 2006, about a decade after one of its cofounders first started taking spin classes at her gym. By June 2019, they had more than 90 locations in North America.[4]

I tried SoulCycle just so I could see what it was all about. Out of all the players in the spin-class space, SoulCycle is especially known for their peppiness, their positivity, and the fact they have so many locations.

When first I showed up, way too early, I discovered that I was actually supposed to be at a *different* location, because Chicago has three SoulCycles within its city limits. (New York City had twenty at mid-2019.) A helpful counterperson got me switched to the right class. Already, I was a failure before I even began.

A few minutes before class, I walked into the room. It was dark and humid, and bikes were everywhere. I found my assigned bike and another helper person adjusted it for me. I clipped in and waited as other spandex-clad people arrived. There were about forty of us, and five were men.

Our instructor, a plucky, skinny, tall woman, came in and got us pumped up and ready to go. This class specifically played 1990s pop jams, and as I am a child of the '90s, I thought it would do well for me to dip my toe into a new exercise method while getting bombarded with music from my childhood.

Did I mention there were candles? There were candles. I don't know if they were real or electric. But they gave the room an otherworldly glow. We weren't just riding stationary bicycles. No—we were on an adventure.

The first thing you need to know about SoulCycle is this: They just kind of throw you in. You don't get much time to adjust, other than knowing there's a knob that you turn left or right to make it harder or easier to pedal. The music starts blasting, the class leader talks into a microphone, and lights start pulsing.

The teacher asked if anyone was new. Only my hand shot up. The class clapped in support of me, and the teacher told me to just watch everyone else and figure things out. That's what I then attempted to do as the music began playing.

I'm thirty-three as I write these words, and I can tell you this: That music was too damn loud. I can't believe I am writing that. My parents were right—I am becoming them. I wish I had brought ear-plugs.

The class started with some basic pedaling. Sometimes we would pop our butts off the seat and pedal to the beat. Sometimes we would go half-time. It would get harder, then easier, then harder, then easier, giving you regular breaks so you weren't going 900 miles an hour the entire time.

Throughout the class, the teacher made sure to tell everyone how great I was doing as a first-timer, and then the entire class would turn and cheer at me. I felt like I was at some sort of positivity seminar, and I mostly wished I was out for a run and listening to a podcast instead.

It was somewhere around Hanson's "MMMBOP" that my legs started to burn. My fitness watch showed my heart rate wasn't going crazy high, nor was I breathing hard, but my legs were definitely not used to this.

The music cycled between faster jams—Spice Girls being a specific joyful moment—and some slower jams, including "Truly Madly Deeply" by Savage Garden, which instantly transported me back to a seventh-grade dance where boys stood on one wall and girls on the other.

I had read ahead and knew to bring water, which I drank constantly. As we neared the thirty-minute mark, my shirt and shorts were soaked. I should've brought a headband, as sweat kept dripping into my eyes.

The room smelled of hard work. Because it was hard. But I also found it to be kind of boring.

Don't get me wrong—I totally get why someone would *love* it. The vibe was supportive. People were having a fun time. And I've never stretched to a Whitney Houston song before, so that was nice. It also didn't have the typical Cro-Mag attitude you get when you walk into some gyms.

But overall, while it may have been fun, I didn't feel like I got as much out of it as I would've by running. I *did* get to revisit some classic jams of my youth, yes. But still, I would've rather been running or on an elliptical or stationary bike at a gym.

MY SOULCYCLE STATS

Let me give you some stats, because I wore a fitness watch and tracked my heart rate throughout. During the forty-eight minutes I was tracking, my heart rate averaged 135 beats a minute, with a max of 173.

If I were training to boost my cardiovascular ability, I'd want to spend a lot of time above 150 beats per minute. According to my watch, I was in that zone for only 18 percent of the total class—or just under nine minutes.

My watch gave me a 2.8 in terms of aerobic difficulty—this means I was just maintaining aerobic fitness. And during that time, I burned 619 calories.

Compare that with a 4.5 mile run I did in a little more than forty-two minutes. I burned 739 calories and averaged a heart rate of 165 beats per minute, with a max of 178.

During my run, how often was my heart in that zone needed to boost my aerobic ability? Almost 96 percent of the time. According to my watch, this was a 4.1 out of 5 in terms of aerobic difficulty, or "highly improving aerobic fitness."

(Of course, this was a run I intended to be hard and long. But I tried to race my ass off in the SoulCycle class, too. It just didn't give me the same benefits, calorie- or cardiovascular-wise.)

We did more than just pedal at different speeds. We changed our pace and moved the resistance up and down, making it harder or easier to pedal. We did a lot of those push-up things with the handlebars. We even lifted some three-pound dumbbells, which became surprisingly hard as hell. You definitely get more of a full-body workout than I would have expected in a spin class.

I also can safely tell you I sang along to Hanson, because I was told to do so by the instructor.

But it's expensive—$30 for two classes at an introductory rate when I tried it, but as of mid-2019 it's $32 a class in Chicago. In comparison, my YMCA membership is $52 a month, and it has stationary bikes. And a pool. And a weight room. And less-peppy spin classes. And so on.

So if you try it, make sure you bring lots of water. And don't get too weirded out by how damn cheerful everyone is.

CrossFit

CrossFit was started when someone who eats rocks for fun and likes getting punched in the stomach as an aperitif wondered, "What if exercising sucked even more?"

You can't be a human being and have not heard of CrossFit. Probably because everyone you know who does CrossFit likes to let you know. It's like that old joke: How do you know someone does CrossFit?

Don't worry—their Instagram will tell you.

That's a dumb joke. But I stand by it as it meets my exacting joke standards. We have fun.

Anywho. CrossFit isn't *exactly* a type of exercise. It's a sport. Anyone who says differently probably has something to sell you. (A CrossFit gym membership, perhaps? Or a membership to their own way of getting in shape.) The end goal of CrossFit is to compete in tournaments and work your way up to an event called the CrossFit Games, which is usually streamed online and sometimes on cable television.

If you check Netflix right now, you'll probably find nineteen movies about CrossFit, and some include the CrossFit Games. I have watched all of them and wish I had abs half as good as the female contestants.

(You don't have to compete if you do CrossFit, obviously. It can be just a good way for you to stay or get in shape!)

Literally, the goal of these games is to prove who is the fittest person on earth. This method of exercising is geared toward pushing yourself in strength as well as conditioning. In the games, people are running long distances, sometimes with massive amounts of weight strapped to their bodies. And then after that, they're deadlifting their weight a hundred times, doing a hundred crazy pullups, and ending it all by swimming half a mile in the ocean or carrying a hundred-pound bag across a football field.

I'm somewhat exaggerating, except that I'm not. Go watch one of those movies if you want some motivation to get off your butt and go for a walk or a run or lift some weights—they always get me going.

Part of the "problem" with CrossFit is that people say it becomes like a cult. Why? Because it's expensive. People talk about it *a lot*. And folks get incredibly dedicated to it. That doesn't mean it's bad whatsoever—sure, you've probably got a few jerks who do CrossFit or who run specific CrossFit gyms. But you've also got jerks who run gyms everywhere. Or who are in every gym. (Looking at you, dude who wears wrap-around sunglasses at my YMCA and the same white tank top that you've written your name in Sharpie on the back as "Swollasaurus Rex" and also hangs weights from your neck and does neck exercises while *still wearing the sunglasses indoors* and tried to fight me because you kept moving equipment I was using because you "didn't like where it was.")

Oh, also, they don't call them "gyms." They work out in "boxes." Because good things come in packages, I guess? At first, CrossFit seemed to be a lot more about marketing and motivation and pushing your limits than anything else. At least those were my initial thoughts. But because I am a *very* talented journalist, I decided to try CrossFit so I could write about it.

First, I researched the CrossFit-oriented gyms in my area. Shocker: They're pretty expensive. After what felt like twelve hours of going through its website, I discovered the price of the one directly across the street from me is $235 a month. But if you're new, you have to sign up for four months no matter what. That's a lot of money to invest before you're sure about something.

Thankfully, there's another gym—excuse me, *box*—that's only a fifteen-minute walk away. The prices there are less ridiculous: $195 for a "Foundations" month, which is all about training you in the basics of CrossFit-style exercises, along with the major barbell moves. Also, through its website, you get 20 percent off. And unlike the other gym's website, its prices were easy to find!

Now, the price drops down to $175 a month after you're experienced. That's still more than three times what I pay to exercise at the YMCA. But unlike the YMCA, I would be exercising in a group setting, with some coaches, doing something probably quite different from what I'm used to. I expected I would push my body more than if I were exercising on my own or working out with a trainer.

THE FIRST CROSSFIT SESSION

For my first session, it was just me and a trainer, who co-owns the gym with her husband. She was pretty easygoing and walked me through *why* CrossFit-oriented gyms train the way they do: It's about using movements that are a part of your daily life, staving off the inevitable decrepitude that happens as we age, and getting ourselves to the highest level of fitness possible.

She was patient while she showed me the various lifts I would be doing that day. Even though I'd been lifting for about three years at that point, she pointed out a lot of issues with my form. The exercises were a lot harder than I had anticipated. At the end of the session, I spent ten minutes doing a set of three things as many times as possible: 50 reps of jumping rope, 10 air squats, and 5 push-ups. I was able to complete the set three times, plus an extra set of jumping rope.

I was pooped after. But unlike how tired I regularly felt after running or lifting weights, I quickly regained my sense of being in control, if that makes sense. During the exercise, I definitely exerted a lot more energy and needed to take more breaks than I would have if I were just lifting weights on my own or going for a fast run. I was almost mad about how much I thought I had pushed myself to be in better shape, only to have that ten minutes of exercise wipe me out.

My trainer assured me this was pretty normal. The day after, I wasn't anywhere near as sore as I had expected. No sore muscles making me unable to walk down the stairs; my arms weren't stuck in a *T. rex* shape. I felt good. And was excited about my next few days of training on the fundamentals.

A MONTH IN

I TOTALLY GET IT AND LOVE CROSSFIT.

A lot of my friends sighed when they heard I was trying CrossFit. It has, well, a reputation of being a bit extreme. And the people who do it of being jerks. And everyone who does it of getting hurt. After a month, it didn't seem that extreme to me. Everyone I encountered was kind, helpful, and supportive. And injuries happen in every sport—I got hurt more training for a half marathon than doing CrossFit. Not to mention, the coaches at my box put a lot of care toward people's abilities, form, and overall well-being.

I had the same kind of misconceptions around Crossfit-style

workouts as I did about other exercise methods before starting this book.

Here's why I like CrossFit:

- It has a community. Most of my exercising pursuits are relatively lonely, especially when it comes to strength-based training. But during my classes, I was surrounded by supportive people who were all there to do the same thing: push themselves.

- A coach watched to make sure my form was good. I hear this isn't the case at every CrossFit gym, but it was at mine.

- Because the workouts are regularly switched, it's a lot less boring than lifting in a gym.

- It's still strength training. I was regularly squatting, dead lifting, and doing other movements that work out all the muscles that I think make me look like a pretty man.

- I wasn't as concerned anymore about what my scale said and was more concerned with my performance. My weight has remained relatively stagnant, but that's fine, as I continue to get stronger and do the workouts faster.

Listen, CrossFit isn't for everyone. And not every CrossFit-oriented gym is made equally. But I was happy I started doing it and bet that I would keep doing it even after this book came out.

FOUR MONTHS LATER
I totally get why people love and continue to do CrossFit-style workouts. But my work schedule changed—I was no longer able to head to the gym at noon and work out unencumbered by technology. (I got a promotion—brag, brag, brag—and had to travel a lot more, which

meant I had more responsibility and it was hard to "plan" exercise when I would get dragged into random meetings all the time.)

It just didn't make sense for my schedule. I had grown to enjoy the camaraderie and the difficulty of the workouts. But it wasn't working for me anymore.

Not only that, but my goals changed. I wanted to be able to run a 10K on occasion but also lift weights and get stronger. While CrossFit is technically supposed to train your cardiovascular ability and get you stronger, I found I barely had the energy to do any training runs.

So I moved to a traditional strength-training program and run three miles or farther at least three times a week. It fits my schedule, and it's substantially cheaper, but I definitely got some foundational strength through CrossFit-style workouts. While they're not for everyone, if you're already active and looking for a challenge, and you've got a lot of disposable income, find a CrossFit gym near you. (I also stopped calling it a box.)

Fun fact: Because of CrossFit, I developed an insane new vein in my arm, not to mention an awesome forearm dimple right next to it. I finally look more like the Disney cartoon prince who resides in my heart.

A (VERY) BRIEF HISTORY OF CROSSFIT

CrossFit officially started as a company in 2000. Its founders sought to combine strength-training with conditioning, high-intensity interval training, Olympic weight lifting, and other exercises.

It's promoted as a physical exercise philosophy and also as a competitive sport. There are thirteen thousand affiliated gyms, most of which are in the United States. One of its big selling points is the "workout of the day," or WOD, which usually involves different kinds of activities.

CrossFit has blown up in recent years, partially because of increased media exposure through the CrossFit Games, the yearly competitions to find the strongest man and woman in the world. And also because, well, a lot of people do CrossFit now. Odds are you know someone who does it. (Don't worry, they'll tell you.)

CrossFit is often attacked because folks say its methods lead to injury. All exercise can lead to injury if you don't do it correctly and safely. The CrossFit-oriented gym I trained at focused intensely on doing each movement correctly to avoid injury.

Delayed-onset muscle soreness

At first, every time I'd go to the gym to lift weights, something terrible would happened the next day. I'd be unable to move.

I would have benched a bunch of weight, maybe used a machine to work my legs, probably done a bunch of curls. I'd feel great, having kicked my own ass and accomplished something. Then I'd go to sleep. Then morning would happen. And then I would try to move anything on my body, and it'd be awful.

This, dear reader, is delayed-onset muscle soreness, better known as DOMS. It's what everyone who starts lifting weights has to deal with. You can't skip it. But I'm here to let you know that not only have you done nothing wrong if you experience it, but also it won't always be like this.

DOMS causes you to feel stiff, can make it hard to walk, and sometimes makes you unable to fully extend your arms. Everything feels sore. And then, on top of that, it lasts for a few days. And many people think they've done something wrong to their body and they stop lifting weights entirely.

This is what I did over and over. I'd join a gym. Go once. Freak out because my body hurt so much. Vow to never do that to my body again.

Nobody taught me that DOMS was normal. And that it didn't mean I'd hurt myself. And that it would go away. And if I worked out again, it would probably go away faster.

See, your body quickly adapts to the stresses you put on it. If you lift weights, it freaks out. But then when you try to lift the same weights again, your body is all, "Oh, okay. We're going to do this a lot? Cool. Cool cool cool. Got it." And then the next time you lift, it doesn't hurt as much. And the next time, it's hurts even less.

If you lift regularly, you get to a point where your body is tired-sore but no longer OMG-life-is-pain-OMG-DOMS sore. You don't get DOMS again unless you try a lift you've never done previously and it causes those new muscular tears to happen in a new way, and your body responds in kind. And then it goes away.

But DOMS becomes a loyal friend. If you stop lifting for a few weeks, it'll come right back. Even if you were lifting a few days every week for years, if you take a break for maybe ten days or two weeks, poof, it'll be back. And then you get to go through it again.

But it also may not come back in full force. I've had times when I've gone a few weeks between workouts because of general life business. When I went back to the gym, I took it easy, dropping the weight down, lifting less than I had the last time I was there, usually doing fewer sets. I'd be sore the next day, but I wouldn't be completely crushed. Then usually by the next workout, the DOMS would be completely gone.

When I was doing CrossFit, because of the constantly shifting types of exercise movements we'd do, I had DOMS a lot more regularly than when I followed a routine. You can get DOMS from different types of exercise, not just lifting weights. Just something to be aware of.

Speaking of routines. You know what group of people follows an *incredibly* specific kind of workout regimen? Bodybuilders. Can't talk about exercise and fitness without bringing that sport (and yes, it is a sport) into the fold.

ANDY'S EARLIEST ATTEMPTS AT LEARNING FROM A BODYBUILDER

I joined a gym while I was living in Florida after college. I was pretty big, well over three hundred pounds, and I'd heard lifting weights could help. I found a big gym and signed up. As part of my membership, I got two free sessions with a trainer.

Enter Chad, my first personal trainer. That's not his real name (or was it?), but it'll do.

When you picture Chad, imagine the shittiest muscle-bound jackass you can. Now give him gelled, short blond hair, a tank top, and a personal bodybuilding website that blasts death metal when you log onto it. Now you have Chad.

Here's the thing: I've always wanted to look like Chad. I want beefy arms, pecs that pop, shoulders that could rip T-shirts. That's how I thought all people who lift weights should look.

During our first session at the gym, Chad asked what my goals were.

"To get in better shape."

He rolled his eyes. "Do you want to get ripped or be a bitch?"

I didn't know what that meant, so I went with ripped. He nodded and wrote something down. Then he asked what I ate. I shrugged and said whatever, just ate anything I wanted.

"Eating is important, bro," he said, then tapped his head. "Willpower. You get me?"

I did not get Chad. I am, almost a decade later, still happy I didn't get him. But I nodded and he took me around the room.

Chadsworth stopped me in front of various machines, explaining which part of your body they would "explode," which was his way of saying "exercise." He assured me his weightlifting technique would help me not only lose weight but get ripped fast. "We're going to trick your muscles," he said. "They won't even know what hit them." He smiled a huge grin, as if this would make sense to me.

It didn't.

To warm up, he had me ride a bike for ten minutes to get me "in the zone." After I was good and zoned, Chaddington had me do a bunch of things on machines, none of which made sense, while he wrote things down on a sheet of paper, which he wouldn't show me at any time. "Secrets, bro," he said, then tapped his head. That's where the secrets lived. (Also, apparently, on his sheet of paper.)

When I neared the end of the reps he'd told me to do on each machine, Chadly would shout and scream that I could do it, that I wasn't a bitch, that I had to finish it. And then I would finish it. He would say, "Good job," and we would move somewhere else.

At one point, Chadder had me lie on my back and try to kick his hand, which he held around his chest, one foot at a time. During my third or fourth kick, I felt some weird sensation go through my back. It wasn't pain, but more like my body screaming, *"What are you doing?"* I listened, and stopped, and told him my back seemed to spasm.

He went, "Uh, okay. This exercise is over then."

We did a few more things, then I went home. He told me he'd see me in a few days for our second session. I stumbled to my car, every muscle destroyed and my soul crushed, if this was what it meant to exercise.

What Chaddy did not tell me, and what I explained earlier, is that the day after the first time you truly exercise is pretty awful because of DOMS. Your body screams at you because of the micro-tears in your muscle you made while lifting weights. (Don't worry—when your body repairs those tears, that's how you get stronger and grow your muscle.)

Guess what? Your body does not like it the first time you do this, as it's a shock to your system. The next day, I couldn't walk. I couldn't straighten out my arms. I couldn't even lift myself onto a toilet when nature called.

I came to our next scheduled workout feeling like the worst. Chad seemed pleased that my body hurt like hell. After another disorienting workout, he then went into his mega sales pitch:

- "Pay me a ton of money up front for a bunch of workouts."
- "Pay me less money but still a lot for fewer workouts."
- "The special thousand-dollars-a-month-on-top-of-everything plan will have me Skype with you and also go with you to buy all your meals for the week."

Basically, Chad wanted me to pay him to become my best friend. He also insinuated he had some "other secrets" to offer me. Judging by his body, and his many posts on his website about how he *was most definitely not* on steroids, I only had one idea what those secrets were.

I decided not to follow up with Chad on his offer of more trainings. I also decided that the gym wasn't what I wanted. Chad ruined it for me. I stopped going to that gym and felt ashamed. I later canceled my membership there.

Chad is bad. Don't be like Chad. Don't train with a Chad.

If you get a trainer and they act like Chad, run away.

ACCIDENTAL PENIS VIEWING, OR THE TIME I WENT TO A BODYBUILDING COMPETITION

The first thing I discovered when attending a bodybuilding competition is that the people competing aren't ginormous. In fact, they're all pretty skinny—they've lowered their body fat so much their muscles pop and glisten under the large stage lights.

The second thing I discovered is that if you go to the dressing room area hours before the event starts and see a sign that says TANNING ROOM and look in, you'll see a completely naked, ripped man, standing in a weird tent-like thing, getting a massive spray tan by a woman wearing a yellow shirt that says KEEP CALM AND TAN ON. Seeing someone hang dong wasn't exactly how I suspected my Saturday to start, but, alas, so it did.

I was at this event for a few reasons, other than accidental penis viewage:

I wanted to talk to some folks who went through the grueling efforts of becoming a bodybuilder. I was thinking, "Hey, maybe I should try to lift like them, just so I can learn more about it, and how hard is it *really*?" (Answer: Very hard.) And:

1. I wanted to see folks at what some might call a peak level of human fitness—the most muscle mass and least fat on their bodies.
2. It was close to my house. (Notice a theme?)

Before I walk you through my day, let me explain how these competitions work. I attended the Windy City Natural Pro-Am, which is a regional competition sponsored by one of the various bodybuilding and fitness organizations, which are governing bodies that decide on rules for the sport of bodybuilding. Just as soccer has FIFA, bodybuilding has its own governing organization.

Folks competed in various divisions, broken down by gender, age, style, and whether they were an amateur or a pro.

I showed up to the competition early in the morning and was given a press pass that had a lightning bolt on it, because I have the power of Thor, apparently.

The theater's audience area was packed with people in workout gear and track suits. Many of them had already lathered up with their fake tans, and most of them wore shirts advertising either the bodybuilding team they were with or some other fitness-related products.

I was reminded of all the show choir competitions I performed in during high school and college. Hundreds of people were in various stages of dress, their hair in different setups, everyone heavily made-up and spray-tanned, people posing to music. Only with much less singing and dancing. (Or so I thought.)

The day started with the head judge, one of seven, explaining the rules, the poses expected, the order in which to do them, and other parts of the stagecraft.

The competitors in the audience were taking notes, asking incredibly specific questions as to how to properly pop a side tricep and other things I would have never thought about.

I quickly noticed something about most of the people here: When they were wearing their jackets and baggy clothes, you couldn't necessarily tell they were bodybuilders.

Brian McCabe, one of the people running the event and the owner of BodySculpt Fitness, a bodybuilding consulting group, had a physique I was envious of. He was in a T-shirt at the beginning, his huge arms sticking out, making me think, "Oh yeah, that dude lifts." The other folks here? It wasn't always clear who was a competitor and who was a spectator.

That's one of the interesting things about bodybuilding: It requires so much hard work, dedication, and soul-crushing decision-making to avoid certain foods and social commitments, but you have to take off your shirt for folks to know you are insanely ripped.

Some folks? You could tell they were ripped. But not *everyone*. I couldn't tell whether some people in the crowd were the competitors or their friends. That's what was so surprising about it.

The goal of bodybuilding is to build as much muscle as possible, then lose *as much body fat and water weight as you possibly can*. It's not so much about actually getting *huge* but about making yourself *appear* huge. And symmetrical.

Before the head judge was done with her opening spiel, she had some parting words, which I think should be on a billboard somewhere: "You're winning because you're here. You probably look the best you ever have in your life . . . but this doesn't define you." In other words, even if you lost, you were still awesome and had achieved so much.

I walked around the theater and backstage area, just to get more of a feel for the event. Here are a few quick takeaways:

- **Every toilet seat looked like someone had murdered a brown M&M.** Everyone is tanned *everywhere*, including their butts, so it gets all over creation.
- **Everyone's trying to avoid touching anything.** Because of the spray tan. I saw folks who stayed in baggy jackets and jogging pants for hours, just so they wouldn't get their gunk on anything and ruin the theater walls or seats.
- **Everyone wishes they could eat or drink.** Multiple times I heard people complaining about their diets of the last few weeks, and most of them hadn't had anything to eat the entire day, nor any water. If you eat or drink water, it can make your body not look as sharp under the lights. Everyone's starving and dehydrated.
- **People are having, uh, other problems.** I overheard more than one person tell someone else how, because of their intense dehydration, "nothing's coming out" (aka no number ones or twos). Because of this, I discreetly took sips from my water bottle throughout the day, lest I make anyone feel bad.

Despite being incredibly skinny, everyone's broad-shouldered. I doubt anyone could have walked side by side down the backstage hallway.

Men have two hairstyles: short or super-gelled. As a balding man, I was happy to see many buzz cuts and much short hair.

Some of the helpers and people at nearby booths were, to put it in such a way as to not get sued, overly giant musclemen. One dude especially looked like he would give He-Man a run for his money. They were much, much larger in terms of muscle mass than those competing in this steroid-free competition. And these people weren't competing. You get what I'm putting down about this *steroid-free competition*? Cool.

You could easily tell the folks competing were getting their bodies through natural means and wonderful genetics. While the amount of food they ate or didn't eat, or how they worked out, or how little water they consumed in the weeks leading up to the competition may not be natural, they didn't get their bodies through, uh, other chemical means.

Everyone competing also had to pass a polygraph test, and the top handful of winners in each category would do a mandatory pee test, to further check for any steroid use. These people looked amazing, but in a way that seemed attainable by us mere mortals.

One guy I talked to was Gary Ramos, a twenty-nine-year-old from Chicago's North Side. He was fit, tanned with as much oil as possible, and had a happy attitude, by far the most smiley person at the event.

Gary told me it was his second year competing in bodybuilding. He was a former collegiate baseball player, and after he graduated, he was looking for a sport he could do that was competitive. Gary was lifting weights all the time already, so he decided to dig into bodybuilding to learn more about the sport. A former personal trainer, he got a bodybuilding coach—which many in the sport have, mind you—and fell in love with it immediately.

"It was a new way to challenge my body and my mentality," he said before the event. "When I step on stage, it's that same feeling as when I played playoff baseball."

It was his pro debut, and we talked a bit about the prep work he'd done before the show. He told me he spent the last month or so eating 30 grams or fewer of carbs *a day*. That's the equivalent of about two pieces of white bread or one Snickers bar. (And now I'm imagining a Snickers bar sandwich, which sounds delightful.)

The night prior, Gary stopped drinking water around six o'clock, and he said his mouth was dry, his lips were chapped, and boy, oh boy, did he want a drink of water.

Even though he was happy about how he looked, he did say there were some downsides.

"I don't feel the best," he told me. "If I get up too quick, I am dizzy."

I want you to know that Gary was wearing some bulky clothes at the time, so I couldn't tell how in shape he was. Later, during the event, I was backstage, attempting to avoid seeing any more naked people, and Gary was giving another, younger bodybuilder a pep talk, still just being the grinniest person in the room.

At this point, Gary had his shirt off. He was in amazing shape. I am not saying this just because he was kind enough to talk to a random chubby guy—me—who was walking around interviewing super in-shape men and women. I am saying this because I was envious of how he looked, even though I knew all the hard work he had put into it was something I never thought I could do.

Gary had clearly worked his butt off—literally and figuratively, or as I like to say, liguratively (please do not cut this great word, editor, unless you think I should have gone with figerally)—and was psyched to compete. I watched him as he made it to the finals, flexing on stage, full of joyous attitude.

But here's the bummer: Despite being one of the most in-shape people out there, and my thinking he was basically the same if not better than most of the other men in his competition division, he still came in ninth—last place.

I caught up with him after the competition. The man was full of joy. He didn't seem too phased by coming in last. Meanwhile, I still remember getting a purple ribbon for last place in a sixth-grade track meet. (Fun day: They didn't even tell us we would be having a track meet. They just decided, hey, sixth graders, we're walking to the high school track so you can go run in your normal school clothes. Good luck!)

Still, Gary had worked hard and achieved his own goal of pushing his body. Just like you, dear reader, can do with whatever you choose to get more active. Now, I'm not saying you need to choose bodybuilding, but you can probably pick some sort of event—a 10K, a strength competition, a bicycle ride for charity—that motivates you, just like Gary had.

I asked him his plans, now that the competition was over. His grin spread across his face again.

"I'm going to get Pequod's," he told me, naming the best deep-dish pizza place in Chicago. (Fight me.) "And then I'm going to get ready for the next competition."

Other bodybuilding tidbits

- One bodybuilder dude came out as a mime and mimed to a song while flexing. It was awesome.
- Another dude came out in a Batman outfit and flexed while music from *The Dark Knight* played behind him. It was also awesome.

- One woman was the only competitor in her division, so she automatically won, and also got a bunch of money!
- Families came to cheer, which was weird hearing parents yell at their kids to flex their butts more. (I only know they were parents because a mom turned to me and said, "That's my son, so this isn't weird." Yeah, no, totally not weird.)
- The toddler daughter of a competitor was near me and, when her dad went on stage, was like, *"That's* daddy?" And her mom was like, "Oh yeah." And then the little girl asked, "Is he coming back when this is done?"
- One competitor in the female bikini competition was sixteen. I felt weird about all the people yelling at her.
- Before the competition, we all stood and sang the national anthem while smoke machines blasted on the stage and made it look like maybe Uncle Sam was about to come out and flex his glutes.
- One person actually said this out loud: "It's a marathon, not a sprint. Put your mind to it and hashtag grind."
- The concession stand was like 90 percent chips, something none of the competitors were allowed to eat until they were done. I didn't buy any. For solidarity purposes.
- During an early round, a man yelled at another man, most definitely a stranger, "You're a bad boy with them lats and delts!"
- "Kids these days just keep getting tighter and tighter," said one man, and it actually wasn't creepy. He was madder than anything.
- Number of times I heard someone shout, "Obliques, bro!": 4

THOSE ABS AREN'T REAL

Now that I just walked you through the strenuousness of a bodybuilding competition, I felt we should talk about abs. You see them in every fitness magazine, in any movie where a superhero takes a shirt off, and at many beach volleyball games throughout the world. It's as if you don't have them, you've failed.

For some people, they've got eight. Or six. Or twelve. And they look so shiny, and the people who have them make it seem as if they're going, "Oh, these old things? They just showed up one day! Ha ha ha, isn't that *wild*?"

Yes, it is crazy. And because of this, so many people think that unless they have popping abs, they aren't in shape. If you ask people who are looking to get in better shape to tell you their goal, many say, "I want bangin' abs."

It's a great goal. But here's the truth: Most of us aren't going to get abs.

I know, I know, this is hard to hear. But it's also good to hear for many reasons·

1. **Not everyone is genetically predisposed to abs.**

    Just as some of us are tall enough to dunk a basketball, some have amazing calves without doing any work (that would be me), and some have the *perfect* kind of wavy hair that's not too curly but not too straight and is just so great, some people are born with better abs. You can't do anything about it. You either have them or you don't. And even as hard as you work out, they may never truly show up.

2. **Getting abs requires losing a lot of fat.**

    Most people don't start to see abs until they're at around 12 to 15 percent body fat in men, and 20 to 25 percent in women. That's *a lot of fat to lose* for most people. While it's definitely achievable, it's also a ton of work. All that just so someone can see your abs, which are usually covered by clothing most of the time? Not worth it to me.

    Not to mention, a lot of times when you see people who

seem super ripped, with gleaming abs and whatnot, they're actually just incredibly skinny. That's great for them, but again, not all of us are genetically predisposed to ever get to that level of thin.

3. Exercising your abs directly isn't always the best.

Depending on who you talk to, many of the traditional ab-oriented exercises aren't the best for your spine, especially if you're using weights and crunching your body.

But many people think this is the main way to get abs—do one hundred sit-ups every day and they'll suddenly appear. Actually, almost every major exercise you do requires you to use your core to stabilize yourself, which includes your ab muscles. Running, squatting, pull-ups, bench presses, walking, hitting a baseball—they all require you to use your core. You indirectly hit those muscles a lot, which means you have less chance of hurting yourself than when you do something that can cause spinal injuries, such as a sit-up or crunch.

4. Those people with abs in photos are faking it.

When I say "faking it," I mean they've probably done a few things before a photo shoot. They've fasted, sometimes for weeks or months, eating low amounts of food, especially carbs. They also dehydrate themselves to an intense degree. Then, before the photo session, they work out their entire bodies, especially their abs, so they pop even more. Then they flex super hard while photos are taken. And then they're done. Years of work, months of struggle, weeks of dehydration for fifteen minutes of photos. Their abs may go away an hour after those photos are taken, so it's not even like they *truly* exist all the time.

Take Hugh Jackman, for example. I read an interview where he talked about preparing for scenes in a Wolverine movie that involved his shirt being off. He's playing a literal genetic mutant with superhuman strength. His veins needed to be ripping through his body, and he needed to look like something unnatural. That meant watching his diet to an extreme degree, like a bodybuilder, and then dehydrating the hell out of himself.

Apparently, he also had to shoot action scenes while in that dehydrated state when all he wanted was some water. Hugh said he was miserable, getting terrible headaches, and had to wait until they said they got the footage before he could drink water and make that barely attainable look disappear. But he's an actor. You're probably not.

5. People with nonstop abs year-round live a super strict lifestyle.

These people have probably been exercising for many more years than you've ever thought. They have their diets on lock. They exercise long hours. And when they go out with friends, they don't eat the occasional piece of cake, or have a beer or a piece of candy. Their lives are, truly, a lot harder than I would ever want mine to be. All so they can maintain their abs twenty-four hours a day. Is that what you want? Probably not.

But if it is, that's cool. Just understand the road ahead of you is long and somewhat miserable, yet still achievable. And you have no clue what your abs may actually look like when you finally make them pop.

6. Photoshop is a thing.

As we've seen time and time again, what is shown to us in popular entertainment isn't real. That includes people's bodies. Magazine covers are heavily edited to make muscles pop, make people skinnier, and make them appear more in shape than they are. Movies and television shows are actually doing live-action versions of this, fixing people's faces, making their muscles appear bigger, and more, all with the click of a few thousand buttons. You shouldn't compare yourself to these people, as, again, it's not real.

■ ■ ■

Here's the big truth about abs: You already have them! If you managed to get out of bed today, that proves you have abs. If you moved in any direction, you have abs. Just because they're not visible doesn't mean that you don't have them or that they're not strong. It's a lot of work to get something quite superficial that you can show off only in certain situations.

If that's a goal of yours, that's great. But it shouldn't be your *only* goal. It should be an extra benefit that happens because of the other healthy choices in your life. A strong core is great because it helps with your mobility, especially as you age. But having visible abs for the world to see while you're at the beach doesn't help you as much in the long run.

Fun fact: Beauty standards change. As I write this, the most attractive kind of man is one who is balding and also has *amazing* calves.

ANDY TRIES BODYBUILDING

After looking at the bodybuilders and watching them get mega-swoll, I decided that I wanted to look better in a T-shirt. I wanted to try the bodybuilding lifestyle, just to see what it would do.

That meant I would probably need some help.

I started my current, long-lasting health and fitness journey without a personal trainer. You might not want or need one. Personally, I don't think most people do. But because many people find success using them, and because I'm aware that I *actually* don't know everything, I wanted to see what using one would be like for this specific goal.

I found a pretty dang good personal trainer who embodies every-thing you should want from one. Not to mention, he's a fifteen-minute walk from my house, which is also pretty great.

His rates are reasonable, and most importantly, he asks what your goals are and then gears your workout toward them.

His name is Drew Swithin, and he runs Golden Physique in Chi-cago.

He's not a meathead, like our friend Chad. He's in shape, he's kind, and he explains why he's having you do what you're doing. More than any other trainer I've met, Drew talks mostly about the importance of eating. If you're not eating right, he says, the workout can only do so much.

Most trainers work with you one-on-one at a gym somewhere. Drew is a bit different. He has his own gym and has you exercise in a group. Everyone works out individually, according to a plan that Drew talks over with them before their workout. Even though a handful of people are exercising at once, the space is small enough for Drew to watch you and correct your form, see if something's too much for you that day and have you switch to another exercise, and to coach you, all while staying upbeat. Unlike instructors in a giant exercise class, he still has time to focus on individuals when they need it.

For an extra fee, Drew offers a bit of life coaching around your meals. He'll email you every week, asking what you've eaten, and you send him back a list, which helps you track your meals. And Drew can tell you about which choices he thinks are better for you and which aren't so great. (He also wants you to know that getting abs is a ridiculous thing for most to focus on, which made me feel good, as that's never been a goal of mine.)

Now, to be honest, after a while, especially when I would go on a binge with some pizza, sending him a list of what I'd eaten bummed me out. Because I knew I was making some poor choices. And Drew knew that I knew better. So that can sometimes suck. But it was nice to be reminded, and he was never scolding about my decisions—just letting me know about some alternatives or what had helped him or other clients in the past.

I talked with other bodybuilders who'd all had similar coaches: people who would check in on their progress, their eating habits, their training. Because bodybuilding is a sport, it makes sense to have a coach.

I wasn't planning on competing, though. My goal was to look better in a T-shirt.

Here's the basic idea around bodybuilding: Instead of focusing purely on strength—the ability to move the most weight at low reps—you focus on the total volume of weight you're lifting.

This is why a lot of strength programs have you doing fewer sets with fewer reps. (Usually these are called 3x5 or 5x5 methods.) In a hypertrophy-oriented program—a muscle-building program—you do more sets with higher reps but lower weight.

If you bench-pressed 175 pounds a rep, for three sets of five, that's 2,625 total pounds moved. The heavier the weight, the more taxing it is, and the more strain it puts on your body.

If instead you bench-press 125 pounds a rep, for three sets of ten, that's 3,750 pounds moved. More total volume of weight. And, perhaps, because it's a lower-intensity kind of exercise, you may not be as gassed by the end of it.

Now, this doesn't mean bodybuilders aren't strong. Far from it. Many still focus on strength, but the overall goal isn't to get as strong as possible. It's to build up your muscles as much as possible. (And the stronger you are, generally the more muscle you have, too.)

Before attending Drew's gym, I'd never done any sort of group fitness. Even though I was working on my own routine, going to the gym became addictive. I felt connected to those around me—

everyone's going through the same sort of pain, and we're all getting help from the same person.

We took some before photos during my first consult. I was training for my first half marathon at the time, which gave Drew pause.

"Which are you trying to do?" he asked. "Look great in a T-shirt or be able to push your body to run a long distance?"

"Both," I said, not knowing that was a dumb answer.

Drew gave me a great explanation, which took more than a year to sink in: The goals were somewhat contradictory. Running and burning so many calories can impact my ability to lift weights and maintain muscle. I'd have to choose, he said.

Because I am very smart and obviously know everything, I just shook my head and said I'd be fine.

Spoiler: I wasn't.

I tried my best to eat like a bodybuilder. I really did. My diet was broccoli and cauliflower and chicken and nuts and cheese and boring, boring, boring. I prepped my meals in advance, making a bunch at once. I ate good oatmeal. I protein-shaked myself into the stratosphere. (It's important to note that Drew hadn't suggested I follow this low-fat, more-complex-carbs, all-protein-all-the-time diet. He did the best he could, but not every student is a good listener.)

But after a few weeks, that sort of eating was just killing me. I was lifting weights three days a week, really pushing myself with Drew's plan—which focused mostly on my upper body, as, let's face it, my legs are *dy-no-mite*—and I was constantly starving.

Because of my running, I wasn't eating enough.

Because of my running, I wasn't progressing with my lifts.

At the end of six months, my body had barely changed. I didn't have bigger muscles. I was just a smaller version of who I previously was. Losing all the weight from running didn't mean I maintained all my muscle mass.

Instead, I lost muscle while losing fat.

Drew was right. If you have a fitness-related goal, you can't half-ass two things, as Ron Swanson says on *Parks and Recreation*. You need to whole-ass one thing. (Also, Drew had suggested I walk instead of doing the endurance training, as that sort of training can deplete your glycogen stores, pushing you toward craving more carbs to fill those stores back up.)

Did I look better in a T-shirt at the end of everything? Not really. I looked more or less the same. Was I stronger? Sure. Could I run a long distance at one time without wanting to die? Sure.

But I had failed at my initial goal—aesthetics over everything—because I wasn't following the steps to achieve that goal. Which is one reason you should make sure your goals and the work you're doing align with each other.

If you're a *real* bodybuilder reading this, you probably think my routine was crap. I should've been in the gym six days a week (which is something I've done in the past, believe me). I didn't dedicate myself to the right things. I didn't eat correctly. And I don't disagree with you, man. Also, nice pecs.

That's why I decided to focus on a new goal: I wanted to get as strong as I possibly could.

STRENGTH-TRAINING HISTORY

Training for strength isn't anything new.

In the sixth-century BC, the Greek wrestler Milo of Croton (what a cool-ass name) was said to exercise by carrying a newborn calf on his shoulders. (Whether this happened, I don't know, as my attempts at time-traveling backward have, so far, been utter failures.)

As the animal got older and bigger, Milo would have to get stronger and stronger to be able to carry its added weight. (This is literally how I train to get stronger at squatting, by the way—except replace the bull with "barbell and weights" and it's the same. Also, less cow poop.)

Sadly, Milo apparently died while trying to rip a tree apart with his bare hands. They got stuck in its trunk, and then a pack of wolves came and ate him.

This is why I stopped trying to split trees apart with my hands. I'm deathly allergic to being eaten by wolves.

Feats of strength have been around through all recorded history and in many different civilizations. The modern sport of weightlifting traces its roots to European competitions in the 1800s.

But the Olympics in 1896 more or less codified the basics of using dumbbells and barbells, and we moved on from there. Now you can walk into any gym in America and see all sorts of methods of strength training, but the fundamentals remain the same.

Lift weight in a prescribed fashion. Then the next time you exercise, do the same thing, except make it harder.

Just like carrying a calf on your back, lifting weights helps you get stronger by making your body work harder.

I think that sums up almost everything you need to know about the images you see in the world of super in-shape people.

ANDY GOES TO WATCH PEOPLE STRONGER THAN HIM

A woman in her seventies made me want to become stronger.

I had been lifting weights for a few years, trying to get stronger over time, of course, but I was never truly focused on strength. I thought I was good focusing on more volume all the time, like my trainer had suggested. I didn't want to *hurt* myself with those super heavy weights. But my friend Bryan told me I should go to a strength competition to see what it's like.

Some people train to run as fast as they can in races; others train to be as strong as possible. You may have seen Ironman competitions on ESPN 17, or perhaps stumbled across a YouTube video of someone bench-pressing five hundred pounds. They're impressive.

Strength competitions are one thing many people use as a goal to push themselves. Bryan told me about the U.S. Strengthlifting Federation Fall Classic happening up in Evanston, Illinois, a city north of Chicago. The chance to see superstrong humans was only a train ride away.

I showed up to the gym early in the morning to watch a few dozen men and women lifting their way to victory. These were people from all walks of life, similar to those in the bodybuilding competition I'd attended. And just as in that competition, a lot of the folks walking around? You couldn't tell if they were competitors or spectators.

Except for the people in singlets—I quickly figured out they were competing. Because those were the people warming up with weights I could lift only in my dreams.

For this competition, they were doing three lifts: the squat, the standing overhead press, and the deadlift. For each lift, you had three opportunities to lift the most weight. Three judges watched each of the lifts—at least two had to say it passed, or else it didn't count. The idea was to push yourself each time and get as much lift as possible.

Lots of threes involved here. It's like the holy trinity, except for strength. (And now we know why Jesus is always depicted as having rock-hard abs. He's swoll for your sins.)

Many of the competitors were hitting personal records with every lift. It was astounding to watch. A few months prior, I had thought about competing, but seeing as I was still recovering from running a race a few weeks prior—this is an excuse, just so you are aware—I decided to watch instead.

Your score is a calculation based on the amount you lifted and something called your Wilks coefficient, which is a fancy way of saying your weight and your age. Everyone was weighed immediately after they finished their lifts, so you couldn't do what boxers do and cut a ton of water weight beforehand so that it *seemed* like you're smaller than you really are.

Instead, it was meant to be more realistic about how much you weighed. The higher your score, the better you did. So one person squatting 300 pounds may get a lower score than someone squatting 275, especially if the latter person is twenty years older and weighed 100 pounds less.

I talked with lots of folks. They all had stories about training—following a strict regimen, focusing on those three lifts, eating a high-protein diet, and sleeping a lot. Almost all of them talked smack about people who run, and the announcers cracked jokes about one of the competitors who ran marathons.

Everyone did feats of strength I thought were amazing. One man I talked to was Michael Coon, a thirty-seven-year-old who looked much younger. He was visiting from Ann Arbor, Michigan, and this was only his second strength competition since deciding to get serious about his lifting about two and a half years prior.

"It just sort of happened organically," he said of deciding to pick up the sport. "It's exhilarating and exciting to get so much stronger so fast when you realize what one is really capable of doing."

Michael was strong. I saw him squat and overhead press huge amounts of weight. But the most amazing thing to me was watching him deadlift 236 kilos, which is 520 pounds in American. That's the most weight I've ever seen a human being lift off the ground, and he made it look easy.

Other people did astounding things. But I think the most important story to tell you is about Ann Buszard, a strength competitor who was seventy-six when I met her.

About a year and a half before the competition, Ann had noticed she was getting weak in her legs, specifically when she bent over to pick things up. Getting out of chairs had become harder and harder. A retired nurse who lives alone, she was getting a bit concerned about her lack of strength.

Her son is a strength competitor, and he suggested a doctor in her area who specifically trains elderly people in basic strength movements. She had never done any exercise in her life, specifically none involving weights or a gym. So doing squats, deadlifts, and presses with a barbell was completely alien to her.

Yet a few moments after we talked, the 143-pound woman was about to deadlift 200 pounds. Deadlifting 200 pounds is hard for anyone, let alone someone in their seventies.

Ann told me she noticed results about two weeks after she started training a few times a week. It was like her body had woken up, and suddenly she was able to pick things off the ground without difficulty.

Weight lifting changed her life, she told me.

"Not only in my stamina," she said, "but in my balance and strength, obviously. And your attitude toward life, especially—it carries over."

We had to cut our interview short because it was her turn to compete. The crowd of lifters roared as she went over and easily deadlifted 200 pounds. The whole place exploded, and she was all smiles.

Lifting so you can compete sounds like a great reason to lift weights. And then you can only hope that someday you'll be as strong as Ann.

ANDY TRIES STRENGTH TRAINING

I'm going to not bury the lede on this one: The best results I've had, in terms of how I felt my body looked and my actual weight when standing on a scale, came from training purely for strength.

I've heard this again and again from friends. They didn't get their best results from running, doing yoga, or anything else. It always came from lifting heavy shit off the ground and fighting against gravity.

Throughout researching this book, though, I got a bit off track. I spent a lot of time focusing on running and neglected lifting. (Sure, my CrossFit-style workouts involved lifting weights, but they weren't focused *purely* on strength.) Guess what happened to my body?

It no longer looked how I wanted it to look. I was at my lowest weight after running my second half marathon, five pounds away from my goal. But I still *looked* chubby. I didn't look like I had that many muscles. I didn't have the look that men and women try to chase because of the media.

Guess what started giving me that look again?

Lifting. Heavy. Ass. Weight.

The best I've ever felt came from lifting heavy-ass weights, too. That's not just anecdotal—science backs me up.

A few studies have shown that adults who focus on strength during exercise—resistance training, as it's called in one study,[5] which is another term for strength training—had significantly reduced depressive symptoms.[6] And you don't have to necessarily go all out and lift so much weight you want to pass out: These mental health benefits came from folks who performed at lower- to moderate-level intensity during their training sessions.

It can also help with anxiety, something I've struggled with for years. There was a point when I was too scared of the outside world to leave my home or be in large crowds. But research shows that strength training is associated with a reduction in anxiety symptoms in healthy adults. (The key word there being "healthy," which may skew the results a bit.)

Still, anecdotally, my friends who lift weights struggle with depression less. When I stopped focusing on running half marathons and went back to focusing on the gym, I noticed a decrease in my sad days. My mood was better.

My self-esteem was also up. The research backs this up, too—in younger and older adults, those who do strength training have improved self-esteem. It also increases the self-esteem in populations dealing with cancer, depression, and cardiac rehabilitation.

After one of my bouts with CrossFit, I decided to try a popular strength-oriented program, StrongLifts 5x5, for twelve weeks to see what would happen. Even when I was lifting previously, it was usually still in the hypertrophy style—lots of volume, not as much strength.

I thought I was strong, sure, but I'd never followed a strict strength-focused program.

(It should be noted, I didn't follow the program perfectly. Two or three days a week, on days I didn't lift, I'd run three or four miles. At the end of each lifting session, I usually did some accessory work focusing on my arms, and I did *lots* of push-ups.)

This program focuses on the "big five" lifts: bench press, squat, barbell row, overhead press, and deadlift. Here's where I started and ended with each, and what I was able to do for five sets of five after twelve weeks.

Bench press: 115 to 175 pounds, a gain of 60 pounds
Squat: 185 to 280 pounds, a gain of 95 pounds
Barbell row: 135 to 200 pounds, a gain of 65 pounds
Overhead press: 75 to 130 pounds, a gain of 55 pounds
Deadlift: 265 to 330 pounds, a gain of 65 pounds

Now, because of my travel schedule, I had a few weeks when I was able to lift only twice at a gym with a barbell. I had one week when I traveled so much that I was able to go to a real gym only once—I had to spend the rest of the time using a hotel gym, which didn't have any of the equipment or the weights I needed to properly exercise.

But did I get unequivocally stronger? Yes, I did. Does my chest look better in a T-shirt? It does. How about my arms? Oh yeah.

My legs still are big, and I've still got a chubby midsection, but it's definitely *thicker*, if that makes sense. Thicker in a good way.

But more than anything, I feel *amazing* because of what I was able to do. Every time I was able to put more than my body weight on my back and squat it, I felt like a god. It also gave me a regular goal with each gym session—try to be stronger than I used to be. Like a video game for my muscles.

I plan on making strength a big part of any future exercise endeavors. While I may not be competing in any strength competitions in the future, I definitely will be trying my best to be as strong as I can be.

Meanwhile, you're probably wondering how I did on that half marathon I wrote about training for, aren't you?

ANDY ATTEMPTS TO RUN A HALF MARATHON (FINALLY!)

The Chicago Half Marathon starts in Hyde Park, goes up Lake Shore Drive, and then heads back down, ending close to the starting line. The Hyde Park neighborhood is known for a few things: the University of Chicago and Michelle and Barack Obama first kissing outside a Baskin-Robbins.

And I had come down here, along with about twelve thousand other people, ready to attempt the longest run of my life.

The race was on a Sunday, and the night before, my then-girlfriend and I went to a neighborhood Italian place. I was attempting to eat lots of carbs before the run, so I would have the necessary energy stores and not hit the dreaded wall I had read so much about. I ate a lot of bread. I ate a lot of pasta. My girlfriend and I wondered how many times the Obamas had eaten there and whether they'd sat in our booth.

That night we stayed at a nearby hotel. The race started at 7:00 a.m., which is dumb, and I didn't want to wake up at 5:00 a.m. just so I could get all the way down there in time. Instead, I paid a bunch of money so I could wake up at 5:30 in a strange bed. I'm a genius.

Anywho, the morning of, I got out of bed and took a shower to wake up. Did some stretches, because my right knee was still kind of pissed at me. Got dressed in my running clothes. I crammed some energy stroopwafel things in my pocket—they're basically fancier and more expensive sugar cookies. During my longer runs, I had been eating one of these about every three miles or so to give me some extra energy from the sugar when I started to hit a wall, and since it had worked before, it would work again, I thought.

After we left the hotel room, I realized my first huge mistake: I almost forgot my nipple guards. I went back and got loaded up. #ProtectTheNips

My girlfriend wasn't running the race because she is smarter than me. She was there for emotional support and, I assume, to remind me how dumb running a half marathon is. We made it to the running area and said our good-byes.

That's when the first bad moment arrived. I had to pee.

The bathroom situation at the starting area of the Chicago Half Marathon was somewhat atrocious. Just a ton of porta-potties and utter chaos. Nobody was happy. Everything smelled terrible. Not to mention, the sun wasn't even up yet and it was already about 50 percent humidity and in the mid-70s.

This day was going to suck.

Twelve thousand people had signed up to run the race, and they were all in front of me in the bathroom line.

While I waited for an eternity to use the restroom, I thought about the horror stories around people, uh, losing their bathroom-holding abilities during long runs. Other than that one time during training, that had never been a problem for me. I was hoping today would be the same. (Is this foreshadowing? You'll have to keep reading to find out!)

All of us—more people than lived in my hometown, mind you—got corralled in different areas depending on the times we thought we would run the race in. Everyone around me was talking about how hot it was. People seemed concerned. I didn't know any better, so I thought maybe they just had the pre-race willies.

The race begins

And then, after a brief countdown, we were off. I've got to be honest: The first few miles felt great. That part of Chicago is truly beautiful, and with the sun just coming out, it felt pretty bodacious to be surrounded by all these other people who were doing the same crazy thing as me—attempting to run 13.1 miles.

Then we turned onto Lake Shore Drive and my whole world became pain.

During my training, I mostly ran in neighborhoods. Where trees are. Where shade exists. Lake Shore Drive is a multilane roadway with no shade, next to the water, and just pure angry asphalt. I suddenly realized this could be a terrible mistake. But I soldiered on, because I had signed a book contract that said I would run a half marathon.

My pace during the first five miles wasn't so bad. I was sticking close to 9:30 minutes a mile, which, as a tall, large man, I felt great about. But at around mile seven, my body started to suffer. I took a break and walked for thirty seconds. I felt I had earned it, you know? Running in the sun on a highway for multiple miles makes you think you suddenly deserve little perks in life.

When I started to run again, my right knee was killing me. Every step was agony. At first, I hobbled along, but then after a minute, either it stopped hurting or my mind pushed the intense discomfort away, realizing I was, in fact, doing this dumb thing and wouldn't be stopping anytime soon.

That's when I saw my first person pass out.

I was running with this woman, about my age. She looked in great shape. We were keeping the same pace, moving along. I turned to see how she was doing, and I saw her stumble, then fall to her knees, then on her back. She started convulsing. Spectators rushed to her side. A thought ran through my mind: "This is pretty stupid and dangerous. That woman appeared to be in much better shape than me. Why am I doing this?"

Because I said I would. I kept running, even though my brain's warnings sirens were starting to get louder.

About every mile, I took a thirty-second break to walk. My lungs seemed to be keeping up with everything; it was just literally my body and legs screaming that I needed to take a breather. I would use those short breaks—which later became minute-long breaks, then "to hell with it, I'll walk as long as I want"—to eat my little energy cookies.

I took every shot of Gatorade and water offered at the water stations. I shoved ice down my shirt and pants. I did everything I could to cool off because, by mile 10, I was in rough shape.

At least another six people, by my memory, passed out near me. I saw a few others seeking medical attention. At one point I saw this beautiful man, who had been running shirtless and had the body of a Greek god, being driven away in a cart. If that guy, who appeared to be the epitome of health, needed medical attention, then what chance did I have?

It's about then that I started to weigh the pros and cons of finishing the half marathon.

Pros of finishing

- I get to say I finished a half marathon.
- My "I ran a half marathon" tweet will probably get a few likes.
- I won't have to say I was unable to run a half marathon in this book where I said I would run a half marathon.
- Nobody can ever take this accomplishment away from me.

Pros of quitting

- The pain stops.
- I can go eat pizza immediately.
- I could still say, "I *ran* a half marathon" and just neglect to mention the part about finishing.

Actual con

- I don't get to tell people I finished the damn thing after spending sixteen weeks training for it.

I decided that finishing outweighed everything else and continued.

It's at about this point that I started giving myself little pep talks.

"Listen, you idiot," I yelled to myself. "You got yourself into this, and you're going to get yourself out of it." At one point I yelled a bunch of swear words and then screamed, "I AM A GOLDEN GOD" for motivation. A woman next to me overheard this and gave me nasty looks.

At mile 11, I wanted to die. I've never felt like that before. Everything in my brain was telling me to quit, to find a way to end this torment. It was terrifying. I can honestly say that I've never been in a position where I felt like I was losing it, as if I would no longer be in control of myself. I knew there was only one thing I could do.

I took out my sweat-encased phone, opened up YouTube, found Al Pacino's "Inch by Inch" speech from *Any Given Sunday,* and hit play.

I'm not necessarily a huge sports fan. But I am a huge inspirational-speeches-in-sports-movies fan. This one is definitely in the top five. (And *definitely* in the top three Al-Pacino–gives-a-long-speech-in-a-movie's-third-act speeches.) To give you some backstory, Pacino's character is a football team coach. They're at the equivalent of the Super Bowl. And it's halftime and they are doing awful. Pacino's character is also doing awful in his personal life. Everything is bad.

Just like how I felt! What fun.

At one point, Pacino's character says, "We're in hell right now, gentlemen. Believe me." Dunno if you've ever started to cry your heart out about two miles from the finish line of a half marathon, but it makes it hard to breathe. I listened to Papa Pacino's words of wisdom, as written by John Logan, Daniel Pyne, and Oliver Stone, and they gave me strength.

My tears turned into strength. (Also, FYI, emotions are good to have.) All of that combined and made me power through. I decided I would run the final two miles nonstop.

But when I had half a mile to go, everything in my tank was gone. I unleashed my final weapon, the only thing that could possibly save me: Bill Conti's "Going the Distance."

Earlier in the week, I had watched the first *Rocky* movie for the first time in probably a decade. I thought, "Hey, someone facing huge odds to do something they never thought they'd do, and they're super handsome and like turtles? Sounds like me." "Going the Distance" is the song played at the end of his fight with Apollo Creed, when they both look like discarded meat Popsicles. And Rocky keeps going.

It's *definitely* in the top three inspirational sports songs of movies featuring Sylvester Stallone.

I played that track nonstop for the final half mile. I saw the finish line. I would be Rocky. I would go the distance. I decided I was going to sprint the rest of the way. Three different people apparently time-traveled from the mid-1990s and shouted, "Run, Forrest, Run" at me. Everything in my body screamed, "Stop!" But I didn't.

Hobbling from the pain, my entire body and mind a mess, I made it across the finish line. I knew my girlfriend was somewhere nearby, and I had to find her, only so I could inform her how stupid everything was. I walked in a daze. Everyone around me had that thousand-yard stare you see in old Civil War portraits.

After the run

My girlfriend was around a curve, behind a partition, super happy to see me. I went in for a hug and immediately began crying again. Using many curse words that I will not include here, I told her, "This was the dumbest thing I've ever done in my life."

I stumbled off, was handed a medal for the run, and then walked into the runners-only area where everyone else aimlessly wandered. Nearby a band was playing classic hits from the 1980s, '90s, and today. They were playing Smash Mouth. Nobody looked happy. Nobody wanted the free beer and hot dogs. Especially not with music from the *Shrek 2* soundtrack.

I walked through the maze that was the finishers-only area, looking for an exit so I could find my girlfriend, who waited somewhere on the other side of the fence, as I had lost her in the haze of Southern California surf-rock jams. After texting confusingly with her, mostly because I had lost the desire to form complete sentences or correct my iPhone's interpretation of my sweaty fingers, she found me in the crowd. We sat on a bench and I cried a little. An announcement came over the loudspeakers: The race had been elevated to "dangerous" conditions, and they were suggesting that people quit. It was, according to my phone, 85 degrees, with 75 percent humidity at the time.

But I did it. I finished the race. It's one of the dumbest things I have ever done. Nothing about it felt good. Nothing about it felt like fitness. It felt like insanity, a bad decision times a thousand. But I did it. And that feels so awesome.

My official time was 2:16:44. According to the website of the race coordinators—who did not answer any of the questions I had emailed about how many people needed medical attention, by the way, because I am an actual journalist and tried to get them to comment on how horrible the race was—about a quarter of those running the race didn't finish. I finished in the top 40 percent of total runners, which means, legally, I am above average.

Fun fact: Lake Shore Drive, where the race was mostly held, is a highway. And seeing as they reclassified the race conditions to dangerous, the road is, technically, a highway to the danger zone.

Second fun fact: Did you know some people regularly run *double* this distance? What the hell are those people thinking?

AND THEN SIX MONTHS LATER ANDY DECIDES TO RUN ANOTHER HALF MARATHON

I ran it in 1:58:04 in 20-degree weather, and it was fine.

Long facts about this short section:

- I thought it would be funny if, after writing about how training for a half marathon is torture and dumb, I tried to do it again, and it turned out it was mostly fine.
- My friends and family said this idea wasn't funny so much as it was "stupid."
- It is less funny when you realize I had to run 303 miles and train for fourteen weeks to make this joke.
- It's not so much a joke anymore, as it is just me bragging about running a sub-two-hour half marathon.
- This is proof that I can absolutely commit to a bit if necessary.
- This time I didn't almost poop myself during training.
- This time I *did* almost poop myself during the actual race.
- I ran faster than Hugh Jackman ran a half marathon in 2011, which legally means I'm faster than Wolverine.
- After running the half marathon, I did a VO_2-max test, which checks the maximum amount of oxygen you can utilize during intense exercise—basically, how good your body is at using oxygen to run fast. According to the test, I was, scientifically, considered above "superior" in terms of my cardiovascular fitness, further proof I am better than Hugh Jackman and have become a real-life X-Man.

- Because I watched my diet more this time, I ended up losing about twenty-five pounds throughout the whole half-marathon training process, but I still do not look like Hugh Jackman shirtless. (You win this round, you Aussie punk.)
- On my first day of training, it was 2 degrees outside and felt like minus 10, so, that was dumb.
- I hid in a porta-potty for forty-five minutes before this race because it was so cold outside.
- I like running a lot, but running a long race during the summer is dumb, and you should maybe not do it.

8

Mental Health and How It Impacts Your Weight (and Beyond!)

CHANGING YOUR BEHAVIOR, ESPECIALLY WHEN YOUR BRAIN DOESN'T WANNA

I first started going to therapy in third grade. I know, I was an early bloomer.

I was an annoying child. There's no easier way to say it. I was bonkers. Running around, causing havoc, my mind running a million miles a minute. Regularly I would forget I was holding a glass of milk in my hand and I'd just drop it.

My parents knew *something* was wrong with me. They just didn't know *what*.

After lots of conversations with professionals who had fancy degrees, they determined I had attention deficit hyperactivity disorder, or ADHD. It's all the rage these days. If any kid is acting weird, they usually get labeled with ADHD and are given some pills.

But in the early 1990s, the prescription from my doctor was cognitive behavior therapy *and* medication. The therapy was the important part. I had to learn to change my behavior and develop coping mechanisms for it.

That's the same way many people need to combat their eating habits—modify their behavior.

All the methods in this book, and in most diet books, are methods of behavioral modification. Where a lot of methods fail, however, is after that initial burst of success. You see change quickly. You think it'll last.

It doesn't. Because you're usually not dealing with the underlying issues. And that usually requires a mental health professional.

In my case, it took me years to discover what my underlying issue was. I was a chubby kid growing up. I was bullied relentlessly for my size. For being smart. For having glasses. For not being the right kind of cool.

(And for later lashing out at everyone and everything because of how terrible I felt about myself *because of the bullying*. Most assholes are created by assholes.)

I was later diagnosed with post-traumatic stress disorder from all the bullying I suffered. Guess how I made myself feel better?

I ate.

When I became a crime reporter in Florida, I spent most of my day covering the lowest forms of human misery in depth. If I talked to someone, it was usually the worst day of their life. Everything around me was tragedy, pain, and awfulness.

Guess how I made myself feel better?

I ate.

Many of us are eating the void, as I like to call it. We use food, alcohol, and other substances to fill whatever is missing inside us. Or to replace what was taken from us.

It wasn't until I was in my late twenties that I was able to figure out some of the underlying issues and work on them. I think when I quit drinking it was the first step to being able to look deep within myself and discover what needed fixing.

This is a long-winded way of me saying two things:

1. Just finding a diet and sticking to it isn't going to lead to success. You need to also modify your behavior and figure out the underlying problems that are leading to the behavior and deal with them.

2. It's okay to seek out professional help, whether it be from a medical professional, nutritionist, or exercise coach.

You're not in this alone.

HOW YOUR BRAIN AFFECTS YOUR BODY

Okay, I said you gotta change your behavior to have results, but it's not so simple, is it? If it were, we'd all just be easily doing it. That's like when someone tells you, "Just stop being sad." Okay, *Greg*. (Or whatever your name is. Probably Greg.)

Before you can start making lasting changes, you probably have to start solving some underlying issues.

Mental health isn't talked about enough when it comes to health and fitness. People just want to say, "Eat healthy and exercise." But if you lack the mental ability to get yourself out of bed, how the hell are you going to make other positive health choices?

Anxiety disorders

More than 18 percent of the U.S. adult population suffers from an anxiety disorder, one of the most common disorders out there.[1] That's about 40 million people over the age of eighteen. I should know—I'm one of them. And I suffer from a couple. (I'm lucky like that.)

I suffer from post-traumatic stress disorder, which various therapists have told me is the result of not just the bullying I received growing up—a lot of it because of my size—but also my work as a journalist. On top of that, I have a generalized anxiety disorder, which sometimes leads to panic attacks.

A little more than a third of folks suffering from anxiety disorders ever receive treatment. For years, I did nothing about my problems. I thought I had them under control.

Not only had I been able to lose a lot of weight, but I was regularly exercising, going to the gym, and feeling great. Then I started having panic attacks. The first one was during a work trip in Seattle while I was eating clams. Then they started happening back in Chicago. Pretty soon I was afraid to be in public spaces.

Do you know how hard it is to go to the grocery store when you're afraid to be in public? It's hard! So instead, I would order in food.

Same went with exercising. Gyms had become scary because gyms had people. Not to mention, I didn't exactly want to suffer a panic attack while I had a few hundred pounds on my back during a squat.

I sought professional help and started seeing a therapist again, but not until gaining back some of the weight I had lost and quitting most of my other healthier eating habits. I still struggle with my anxiety. It ebbs and it flows.

But because I'm working on my mental health, I know the signs when anxiety is getting the best of me.

You know what else is annoying? Exercise has been shown to help with anxiety and depression. But both mental illnesses can make you inoperative, not want to leave the house, or—as I like to do—want to put yourself in a pizza coma.

When I'm on the couch watching Netflix, the outside world can't hurt me, or so I tell myself. Instead, that's why developing healthy habits—and a support system of professionals, friends, family, and others—is one way to help me claw myself out of the couch monster I constantly want to be.

Depression

Depression is something that I haven't been diagnosed with, although I've had a few therapists tell me I have teetered on the edge of it. Folks who develop depression often have a history of anxiety disorders —nearly 50 percent of folks diagnosed with depression are also diagnosed with an anxiety disorder—so it's something I'm constantly on the lookout for in my own life.[2]

There are different types of depression. And depression in general affects people differently, depending on gender and age.

- Depressed men are often more tired, irritable, and angry. They're more likely to show reckless behavior, such as abusing alcohol and drugs. And they usually don't recognize what's wrong with them, so they don't get help, leading to the plots of many detective novels.
- Depressed women tend to feel sad, worthless, and guilty.
- Young children who are depressed tend to refuse to go to school, worry about their parents' deaths, and get anxious when they aren't with their parents.
- Depressed teenagers generally have substance abuse problems and eating disorders.

In 2016, more than 10 million adults had a major depressive episode that led to severe impairment—meaning it disrupted their lives in a major way.

Depression affects women much more than men—8.5 percent of women have depression, compared with 4.8 percent of men.

You may be wondering, what does this have to do with health and fitness? Well, just as with anxiety disorders, issues that affect your mind, such as depression, can affect your ability to properly function or to follow through on plans.

The World Health Organization wrote in a report that depression is the number one cause of disability in America.[3] In Europe, it's the third largest, after heart disease and stroke. It can be and is debilitating for a lot of people.

And it makes me mad to see how folks who are depressed and

overweight get treated. Folks sometimes say the worst things: "Just cheer yourself up and get to the gym!" "It's all in your head, so can't you just think it away?" "Buck up, you'll get through this and then you'll be all better."

You can't think yourself back into happiness any more than you can heal a broken arm by thinking. Many times you need not only a professional's help but also lots of time to heal the underlying problem.

Until you deal with the larger problem—perhaps some past trauma in your life or a substance abuse issue you need to work through with therapy, or it could just be that your brain is wired differently—some of the corollary issues won't be fixed.

Obese people have a 20 percent higher risk of depression, one study found, and for white college-educated people who are obese, the risk of depression rises to 44 percent.[4] What isn't exactly known, however, is which one generally comes first.

As someone who used to weigh a lot more than I do now, I can understand why. I was made fun of my entire life for my size. People would yell at me on the street, letting me know I was fat. I remember once someone went out of their way to call me *fat* Seth Rogen, as the actor had lost a lot of weight at the time.

That shit hurt. I know it hurts for others I've talked to. And we have a society that tells us to keep it inside, to stay strong. And then when folks resort to destructive behaviors—eating unhealthy amounts of food, substance abuse, and other coping mechanisms—after years of keeping it inside, who can blame them?

The research shows that folks who lose a lot of weight tend to have substantial improvements in their depression. (It's especially seen in folks who have surgeries that diminish the size of their stomach, such as bariatric surgery, which can lead to a huge weight loss.)

Our society puts such a standard on size as beauty. And people who don't fit those standards are made to feel like shit about it.

If you think you are suffering from anxiety, depression, or any other mental health issues that could be affecting your ability to function, seeking professional help is a good first step. Only when we start fixing the bigger problems can we think about working on everything else.

MENTAL HEALTH DRUGS

Here's another fun part about dealing with your mental health: A lot of the medications explicitly meant to help with it lead to weight gain. According to one scientific review, "A majority of the psychiatric medications are known to generate weight gain and obesity in some patients."[5]

Ha, ha, ha. It's like you can't win.

Because of this, it can also lead to patients not wanting to continue with the treatment. Also, gaining weight can create *more* psychological problems that need to be addressed. It can be like battling a forest fire with other fires, only to have the new fires get out of control.

This is one explanation why in recent years mental health professionals are a bit less likely to hand out pills to treat issues than they used to be.

It's also why if you decide to use any sort of medication to help with any mental illnesses, you need to see how it affects your weight.

One in nine Americans reported taking antidepressant medication in the past month between 2011 and 2014, according to a 2017 survey.[6] Three decades before that? One in fifty.

Part of the reason is that many of the antidepressants folks use regularly today didn't exist thirty years ago. They're called selective serotonin reuptake inhibitors, or SSRIs. And because this type of antidepressant has fewer life-threatening risks than the drugs used previously to treat similar issues, they started to get prescribed more.

This increase in medication over time isn't because more people are depressed. Instead, researchers say, it's because doctors now give out this sort of medication for other issues, such as sleep disorders, anxiety, and neuropathic pain.

Another study says that one in six Americans takes a psychiatric drug during the course of a year, but that also included sedatives, antianxiety medication and antipsychotics, as well as anti-depressants.[7] Regardless, a lot of people use medication to treat mental illnesses.

So, we've got more Americans taking drugs that lead to weight gain at the same time we've got more Americans gaining weight. While correlation doesn't mean causation, it's definitely something to think about.

Other than the Adderall that I was prescribed as a kid to treat my ADHD, I've never been on any other medicine to treat my mental health issues. (A few times it got close enough where I almost wanted some antianxiety medication, but I decided the side effects weren't worth it.)

I do have friends who regularly take antidepressants, though. Many are overweight, and they say they were less fat before they got on the medication.

I'm not anti-medication. I think it's more important to be able to get out of bed and function than anything else, which these medications can help with. Just know the weight-related side effects that can come into play when dealing with mental health issues.

DRUGS IN OUR DRINKING WATER

Medications, including antidepressants, are ending up in our drinking water in trace amounts. While officials have said they don't believe this could be impacting people, studies have shown that it's impacting some fish populations.

Long story short: Even if you don't want to be taking psychiatric medication, you may be regularly ingesting a little. Time will tell how this has affected our communities.

FIXING YOUR CRITERION VELOCITY

Your brain is a judgmental asshole and sometimes it pushes you to fail.

There. It's out in the open. Your brain is sometimes your own worst enemy. And it's all because of this random function of our minds.

It's called the "discrepancy reducing feedback loop," and it's the reason we get mad when things don't go our way quickly.[8]

Think of it as a judge sitting in your brain who's always paying attention to whatever your goal is, and how much you're investing in that goal, and how much progress you're making.

Let's use the example of going to the grocery store. The judge knows how much you're investing to get there (in this example, the time it's taking) and the progress you're making (whether you're done shopping yet and back home on the couch).

The problem is, your judge has *strong opinions*. It thinks this grocery trip should take thirty minutes. This strong opinion is known as your "criterion velocity."

As you work toward your goal, your judge is judging everything. Okay, traffic is light, so we should get to the grocery store fast. You quickly found a cart. All the avocados are perfect. Hooray! Success!

Your judge is happy and makes you feel good.

But then imagine what happens when you go to the checkout aisle. There's only one lane open at 6:00 p.m., and it's packed with people. You start to feel frustrated, maybe a bit angry, right?

And I bet this happens: Your brain tells you to quit, escape, this is no longer worth the time you're putting toward it.

Now your judge is saying your goal is no longer attainable. That goal is now impossible and the judge wants you to give up and throws you into an emotional tailspin. You get angry!

Ever wonder why you get so irrational when things don't go the way you thought they would? This is why. Your brain judge is making you impatient and it flips you into overdrive.

And perhaps you say, "To *hell with it*," leave your cart, and head to your car, and your brain develops a new goal: Find something to eat—fast.

McWenKingBurger Del Burrito Buffet is down the street. Your judge does some calculations, and now you've got a newer, easier goal.

This is why your best-laid plans get chopped to pieces. It affects not only small goals like grocery store visits but bigger ones, too.

Let's say your goal is to lose weight. Your judge gets fixated on this, starts to come up with its strong opinions, tells you how things should or shouldn't work.

(Sometimes these opinions are based on faulty information—go to any supermarket and you'll find ten magazines near the checkout about how people lost 912,373 pounds in just twelve minutes with this ONE NEAT TRICK. You get the point.)

As soon as you stray from what your judge decided on, you want to quit, give up.

This happens to us all. But there's a way to fix it, and it's what has worked for me and a lot of other people.

Change the goal

The first thing you can do is change your specific goal. Instead of losing thirty pounds, why not make the amount much smaller? When I decided I was going to actively attempt to lose weight, my goal wasn't thirty pounds.

It was five.

Then I would hit that goal and make a new goal of five pounds. I just kept doing this until I got to a weight that seemed reachable.

Later, I changed my goals from losing weight to something else: adding strength. How strong could I get?

Later, my goal was to see how far could I run without stopping. Distance training.

Many times I switched goals because I had wanted to quit. Or in many cases, I *had* quit and felt like a failure. So instead of making it a failure, I instead came up with a new goal, telling myself that I just course-corrected.

Change how much you're investing into the goal

You can do this either with the effort or the resources you're using. Over the past few years, I have often spent too much time focused on health and exercise.

Now, was some of it so I could write this book? Yes, it was. But at other times it was because when I wasn't hitting my goal with all my hard work, I would get mad.

Instead, I lowered the amount of energy I was investing and thus told myself that meant I should be totally fine with a slower pace of progress. And then my brain adapted, and it was fine.

At one point, I was running five days a week, lifting three days, and doing a group class four days a week. Yeah, a lot of days I exercised multiple times. This was all on top of a full-time job, spending time with friends, and writing this book. And then I wondered why I felt like crap all the time.

My exercise regimen is much more manageable now, because I've lowered how much I am investing into my goals.

Change your criterion velocity

Your judge will sometimes tell you how long it should take to achieve your goals, and if you don't hit them in that time frame, your brain gets frustrated. Instead, you should try to override that judge by writing down what your plan is and making sure that it's achievable.

I do this all the time. Instead of thinking it should take twenty minutes to get somewhere, as my brain thinks at first, I usually double the time. I reset expectations for myself.

Then, if I take thirty minutes, my brain goes, "Woohoo! We actually did it faster!" But if I take the full forty minutes, I'm not as mad. That was my expectation.

The same thing was true with my weight loss. Instead of focusing on a number given by lots of professionals—that losing one pound a week is about the healthy limit for most folks—I focused on half that number.

Half a pound a week. If I did more, great. If I did a little less, also okay. But it would all average out.

And it did!

You gotta choose your own goal

The goals we are taught in our society are usually something we didn't get to choose. We were *told* the goal is to be super skinny. We were *told* the goal is to get hella ripped.

We were *told* our bodies should look this way, not that way—no, like this. Every day, our culture directly and indirectly pushes that you're supposed to look a certain way, feel a certain way about your body, do certain things to make it live up to someone else's standards.

And that if you don't measure up, then you're a failure.

To hell with that.

It's not easy to change this conditioning—believe me, I fall prey to it every day. (See the section on weight bias to learn more.) But you can start to make smaller changes in your own life—specifically by deciding what your goals are and *how* you want to achieve them.

YOUR STRESS BUCKET

Think of your body and mind as a big bucket with a small hole in the bottom.

All your life's stresses—your job, the bills that are due, a cold you're getting over—are like water being dumped into the bucket. The bucket can take a good amount of water, sure, and it all slowly trickles out the hole.

But if you put too much stress into your bucket, faster than it can drain, then it'll overflow. That's what gets people really out of whack.

The pressure of finding time to exercise adds water into the bucket. So does going through rough emotional patches, either through your job, your relationships, or just, you know, reading the news about the hellscape that is our modern world sometimes.

All of that impacts you. And if you overdo it, the water will overflow and affect other parts of your life.

Even if you've been doing great with your health—exercising regularly, eating healthy, getting a good night's sleep all the time—you may have a nearly overflowing stress bucket and not know it.

Then suddenly a big work project comes into your life. Or maybe a family member gets sick. Or you go through a breakup.

All that added stress can throw everything out of whack, and you may need to take a few other things out of your stress bucket so you can handle the new issues.

Don't beat yourself up if you realize you've taken on too much. Or if you're not seeing the results you want fast enough. Your body's doing its best to drain that bucket. Sometimes you just need to go easy on it.

WEIGHT BIAS AND HOW IT IMPACTS YOUR MIND

Before I started writing about health and fitness, I had never before heard these two words: "weight bias."

But I had definitely been experiencing them all my life. And it's impacted me in ways I still can't fully fathom.

According to researchers, the basic definition of "weight bias" is this: "negative weight-related attitudes, beliefs, assumptions and judgments toward individuals who are overweight and obese."[9]

Someone giving you a dirty look because you take up a lot of space on a bus? Weight bias.

A television show talking about obesity showing pictures of overweight walking people with censored faces? Weight bias.

Your doctor telling you all your tests show that you're perfectly healthy, but you could still lose fifteen pounds? Weight bias.

Weight bias is incredibly common. Have you ever heard someone—or you yourself—comment on the weight of a stranger or a celebrity? Have you ever experienced someone calling you fat or being shamed about your weight?

I remember once overhearing a guy in the gym laughing at an overweight man for being there. "Look at that fatty," he told his pal, who had his T-shirt sleeves cut off (obviously). "What's he trying to do?"

HE'S TRYING TO BETTER HIMSELF, YOU SHITBIRD.

Weight bias has been associated with higher anxiety, lower self-esteem, more stress, and depression, not to mention body-image issues. If the whole world is constantly telling you that your physical shape is *wrong*, you're going to feel bad about it at some level, no matter how hard you try to cheer yourself up.

And shaming people doesn't even work. They've done studies on it; instead, it can lead to eating disorders, compulsive exercising, binge eating, and other unhealthy behaviors.

It can also make people *not* want to exercise in public because they're ashamed of their bodies. (This is why I started by lifting weights in my apartment. I didn't want to go to a gym and feel judged by people like the dude-bro a few paragraphs back.)

We also internalize this sort of weight bias—people can start to believe they *deserve* the stigma and shaming because it's *their* fault that they *chose* to be fat. This whole book is about how complicated obesity is, and how so much of it is out of our control. But because of weight bias, people internalize these terrible things and it doesn't help them.

Studies have shown that public health campaigns that don't focus on obesity or how overweight you are, but instead promote healthy behaviors that don't relate to one's body size, are actually more motivating.[10]

What a shocker: *Being not shitty to people makes them want to do things!* It's almost as if what you learned in kindergarten is true: You should treat others with respect.

That's why I've tried to make the point throughout this book that you shouldn't try to lose weight to improve your appearance, and that thinness *does not equal* beauty or health.

Promoting weight loss as the way to achieve these already-skewed beauty standards makes people think about their weight too much, which leads to the other issues I've already mentioned in this chapter.

Instead, that's why in this book I focus on thinking about improving your fitness and what you can do with your body, as opposed to its overall shape. If you *want* to lose weight, that's fine, but you shouldn't feel like it's necessary because someone told you to, or society tells you to.

You should make changes because *you* want to. (And because that internal desire is what will lead to your eventual success!)

Interview with an advocate

To learn a bit more about weight bias, I talked with Patty Nece, who does talks with the Obesity Action Coalition, the organization dedicated to combating weight bias and educating the public on it, which you may remember from earlier in the book.

Patty Nece has long struggled with her weight.

"I've had obesity since forever and don't remember a time when I didn't carry excess weight," she told me. "You try different techniques, you do diet after diet, years and years and years."

She carried her weight into adulthood, and her obesity grew more severe as the years went on. And all the while, as a teenager and then as an adult, she was ridiculed for her weight.

Strangers yelling at her as she walked down the street. People making snide comments as they saw her approaching. The same sort of stigma many overweight people encounter every day.

"It didn't matter how many successes I had in all of my life," she said. "Nothing overcame the shame and guilt associated with my weight."

It wasn't like she hadn't tried to lose weight, she told me. She had. (This is a big misconception about those of us who are bigger, by the way. We know we're big. We've tried a lot of things. It's not easy, as the *entirety of this book* has shown you.)

At one point, just like many obese people, Patty experienced something she called "diet fatigue" and she wanted to give up.

"You can only hit your head against the wall a million times, and at a million and one, you ask, 'Why do I keep doing this?'" she told me.

That's when she found a physician who was an expert in obesity. And a big piece of the puzzle that Patty had to solve for herself was to work on the damage that the bias and stigma had caused and how deeply she had internalized it.

During our phone interview, hearing her talk about this is when I started to tear up. I hadn't ever really thought about how much shame I felt about my body—the shame I feel even as I type this—because of what others think.

I realized Patty's story was very similar to my own. Just like me, she hadn't realized there was this thing called weight bias. And just like me, she had to first learn to love herself, to push away the negative thoughts, before she could make changes that lasted.

"If you're internalizing incredibly negative things about yourself, where is your impetus to change or make any behavior changes?" she said. "It's a constant daily battle to remember I'm not a failure. That I'm not worthless. That I am a confident woman who has many successes in her life, and has gotten somewhat of a handle on her weight. Not totally—some of that is out of my control."

Patty said the idea of feeling good about herself had to come first for her. She doesn't necessarily think that should be the case for everyone to start to make changes, but it's what worked for her.

It's what's worked for me, too. About five years ago, after I cut booze and a lot of unhealthy food out of my diet, I was able to start liking myself again. The person I saw in the mirror was someone I enjoyed.

I liked how I was changing my behavior and treating others with more respect. I spent more time volunteering, helping others out, giving back. It made me feel good. It also made it easier for me to keep following my healthy habits.

Patty mentioned willpower a lot during our talk. That so many people equate the ability to lose weight or to somehow *not* become obese with self-control.

The issue is, as I've explained in this book, your body, your mind, our food choices, and everything else about our society have been engineered to make us fat. So it's not just a lack of willpower.

"Willpower is when somebody else calls you a big fat whale or makes *moo* noises at you and you keep walking. That's will-power. Trying diet after diet? Willpower. It's not an absence of willpower. Because it's not all within our control."

Patty told me she does think that some personal responsibility is involved when people become obese—but to look at the world around us and how it contributes to a lot of consumption issues. I told her that most of my research shows how much of this is out of our control, that the world is geared toward making us fatter, and that we're not educated well enough on healthy diets or how to exercise.

She agreed with that basic idea and then told me a story. Patty regularly gives talks to medical students to help combat weight bias and educate doctors to not make assumptions based on a patient's size.

In one of her talks, she asked students to imagine she had just walked into their office. What things would they assume off the bat?

Students called out: *You have diabetes! Hypertension! Your choles-terol levels are bad! You eat too much! You never exercise!* All stereo-typical things that larger people hear on a regular basis, especially from doctors who haven't done a full battery of tests on a patient.

She told them the truth: She doesn't have diabetes. They *wish* they had her good cholesterol levels. She probably eats less than everyone in the room *and* goes to the gym more than they do, too.

Sure, her blood pressure is a bit high, despite all her weight loss and regular exercise, but otherwise? Their assumptions are widely off base.

All this goes back to educating people about weight bias, she said. Not just medical professionals—everyone.

"Until you've experienced it," she said, "or have a close friend who has, you just don't know."

THE INTERNET, SOCIAL MEDIA, AND OTHER THINGS THAT IMPACT OUR SELF-IMAGE

Let's point out the obvious: Social media is a lie.

Nobody's having as much fun as they say.

Nobody looks that good all the time.

It's a lie.

Okay, now that we've gotten through that, let's talk about how social media impacts how we view our bodies.

In one survey, 88 percent of women said they compare their bodies with those they see on social media. Not only that, but half of those women say the comparison is unfavorable.[11]

For men, only 65 percent said they compared themselves with images on social media, and a little more than a third—37 percent—say that comparison is unfavorable.

What's most striking about this survey is that for men and women, health and looking in the mirror are near the bottom of what influences how they feel about their bodies.

Which goes again to the main point: Many of the images we see on social media aren't real. And yet we continue to compare ourselves with them.

That same survey said that 51 percent of women between the ages of eighteen and twenty-four felt pressure to look perfect on social media. And 60 percent of women from *all* age groups said they would post a photo on social media only if they loved how they look in it.

Social media is also addictive as hell. Let me ask you this: How often, while reading this book, have you checked your phone to look at social media? Now that I've mentioned your phone, do you *want* to check social media?

The answer is probably yes.

And what do we see on social media a lot of the time? People with perfect bodies who are living perfect lives, and doing so effortlessly.

Have you ever felt bad because of how someone else was living their life? Have you ever thought, "Dang, I wish I looked like him/her" and then felt bad about yourself?

Yeah, that's why social media isn't the best when it comes to your self-image. And that can add more stress to life, which, in turn, can make it harder to love your body or make progress if you're trying to change.

This happened to me a lot. I would see some fitness dude post a photo on Instagram, and I would research everything that guy did to look like that. And then I'd be mad at myself for, you know, not having lived that guy's life in its entirety.

The thing I have to always remind myself is I'm living *my* life, not someone else's. Whatever I've done to get me where I am, I can't change anything in the past. I can only start to make better decisions going forward.

And just seeing someone who looks bonkers-great on the internet doesn't somehow mean I am doing poorly and that I should quit my healthy habits or think I'm already a failure.

Social media addiction

Here are some behaviors to look out for if you think you may have a problem with your social media usage, according to *Psychology Today:*[12]

- Do you spend a lot of time thinking about social media or planning to use social media?
- Do you feel urges to use social media more and more?
- Do you use social media to forget about personal problems?
- Do you often try to reduce your use of social media without success?
- Do you become restless or troubled if you are unable to use social media?
- Do you use social media so much that it has had a negative impact on your job or studies?

If you answer *yes* to all these, or a lot of them, you may want to seek the help of a mental health professional.

A few years ago, I installed an app on my phone that tracked how much time I was using different apps. I didn't think I was on my phone *that* much, but I had noticed I kept not being able to find time to do all the things I wanted to do in my life.

The results were astounding. I was spending more than four hours on just my phone a day—*a day*—on social media: a mix of Facebook, Twitter, Instagram, and Snapchat. That very day, I deleted the apps from my phone and put blockers on my computer so I couldn't look at them.

I did a cold-turkey detox, which was incredibly hard. I often reached for my phone, wanting to check Twitter, to make funny jokes, to share a photo of something silly I saw in the world. It was hard.

After about two weeks, friends started emailing and texting to make sure I was alive. I hadn't done one of those "I am quitting social media!" posts, so many were rightfully concerned. I told them my story, and many totally got it.

Do I still check Twitter sometimes? Sure, but not regularly. I don't use other social media networks, but even when someone shares a link to something on one of them, I find myself quickly dropping into my old habits, wanting to look at everything and click, click, click.

That's because they intentionally make these apps addictive. (I should know—as a journalist who also is a web developer, I have been trained in *dark arts of making people click and read*, so I am aware of what other programmers do.)

But I have to remind myself how much less stress and anxiety I have now, and how many fewer body-image rabbit holes I go down because I'm no longer constantly on social media.

That and, you know, I have time to write and research books on health and fitness.

The internet is for porn

If there's one thing that I think has also contributed to warped body images, it's definitely porn.

This may seem like a slightly taboo subject, but if we're discussing body image, we should be discussing one of the biggest places people get a warped view of what a "normal" body is.

Let's go over some of the facts first. People watch porn. A *lot* of people watch porn. One recent study showed women watched 1:14 more minutes of porn than men did, though most studies I found showed that men were bigger porn consumers.[13] In any event, with the internet being in the pocket of most people, it's clear that it's easier than ever to find porn.

And it's starting early, too. One study in the U.K. said that 53 percent of boys ages eleven to sixteen had seen explicit material online, and almost all of them (94 percent) before they turned fourteen.[14]

While I know there's a lot to say about how this impacts people's views of sexuality, I think it's also important to note how this affects our views of our own bodies. Vivian Diller, a psychologist who is a former model and dancer, wrote this in *Psychology Today,* which sums it up nicely:

> I believe the distorted, enhanced imagery burdens teenage girls with unrealistic expectations about beauty and body image and with damaging ideas about what is attractive and sexually appealing to others. From the perfect waif-like models in teen magazines to the perfectly voluptuous ones on internet porn, the common theme is that these body shapes are unrealistic and unattainable.[15]

Often, we discuss body image in porn with how it relates to women. Less often discussed are the male bodies, and I'm not talking about, well, their appendages.

Modern porn has ripped men with muscles galore. Just like their female counterparts, these male bodies are often relatively unrealistic and unattainable.

Repeatedly being shown these images, especially when they're mixed in with sexual gratification, has to be distorting our views of what a normal human body is. I know it has for me. (Yes, I've watched porn. And especially when I was exposed to it at a young age, I thought that I had to be a super ripped man for women to want to sleep with me. So I know it's affected at least *one* guy that way.)

Porn, just like other forms of media, has distorted our views of what a body can be. We just need to know that what we see isn't real—for many reasons—and to not judge ourselves accordingly.

"IT'S ALWAYS SUNNY" WHEN YOU LIVE A STRICT LIFE

Rob McElhenney is one of the creators and stars of the TV show *It's Always Sunny in Philadelphia*. He plays Mac, one of the show's lovable sociopaths.

And as a goof for the seventh season of the show, he thought it would be funny if he suddenly gained fifty pounds, because in most shows people get better looking as the series progresses. The whole season had a lot of jokes about him "cultivating mass."

He lost the weight by the next season, and that was that.

Except for the thirteenth season, he decided to go the other way: get absolutely ripped.

(Which, just to be clear, meant lowering his body fat and maintaining his muscle mass, just like a bodybuilder.)

Rob posted a photo on his Instagram, with his fifty-pound-plus version on the left and his super-svelte Greek Adonis version on the right. And then he wrote this, which sums up the lengths one needs to go to have and sustain a body like that:

"Look, it's not that hard. All you need to do is lift weights six days a week, stop drinking alcohol, don't eat anything after 7 pm, don't eat any carbs or sugar at all, in fact just don't eat anything you like, get the personal trainer from *Magic Mike*, sleep nine hours a night, run three miles a day, and have a studio pay for the whole thing over a six- to seven-month span."

In case that didn't drive the point home, he added:

"I don't know why everyone's not doing this. It's a super realistic lifestyle and an appropriate body image to compare oneself to."

I think that sums up almost everything you need to know about the images you see in the world of super in-shape people.

9

The How-To Part of the Book

YOU CAN'T OUT-EXERCISE YOUR DIET

If you want to change your body, first you gotta change how you eat.

Throughout the entirety of this book, everything has pointed to one overriding fact: Behavior modification is mandatory if you want to get healthier. And you've got to keep at it.

Armed with all the knowledge from the other chapters about diets (remember: all of them work as long as you make it your *new normal*), here's what you should do:

You should figure out what diet plan you want to follow, come up with some rules for yourself, and then write them down. It can be a mix of when you'll eat (fasting during parts of the day), whether you'll follow a specific diet (vegetarian, paleo, pescatarian, whatever), and what your goals for following this plan are (to lose weight, gain more energy, build muscle mass, sleep better). Then come up with your exercise plan. Now. . .

■ Figure out how many calories you need in a day based on calculating your total daily energy expenditure, or TDEE, which you can figure out by searching the internet for a TDEE calculator. It uses your personal stats and your activity level to estimate how many calories you burn in a day.

- Come up with a handful of easy meals you can make that contain a high amount of protein and fats, and fewer refined carbs.
- Regularly prepare those meals, and have some healthy, low-calorie snack options that you can mix in, so that you can stay under your TDEE.

If you need more specific options, pick something from each column for every meal, and that'll get you closer toward eating healthy:

Protein (fullness)	Fats (energy)	Carbs (energy and fiber)
Chicken	Nuts (almonds, cashews,	Asparagus
Fish*	walnuts)**	Beans
Turkey	Cheese	Broccoli
Eggs	Avocados	Cauliflower
Lentils	Eggs	Spinach
Seitan	Yogurt	Tomatoes
	Flax and chia seeds	Bananas
		Oats

*Salmon, tuna, cod, haddock, flounder are good. Odds are, if you're cooking fish, it's going to be healthier than grabbing a fast food burger, so don't be *too* concerned with the kind you get.

**These are among the best nuts to get your fats from. That doesn't mean you shouldn't eat others if you think these three are yucky.

Now, I'm not telling you how to cook these things. One, because I am a boring chef. And two, because you'll find more success making food that tastes good to *you*. (You likely do not have the same boring Midwestern palette that I do.) Feel free to use salt, pepper, hot sauce, whatever. Cook it in olive oil, coconut oil, or other oils made from vegetables. Make it tasty.

But if you stick to using one or two things from each column as ingredients in your meals, you'll be surprised at how few calories they'll be, depending on how you prepare them. It'll take a lot more food than you expect to actually hit a large number of calories.

You'll feel full. You'll have more energy. And you'll be shocked at how quickly you can learn to whip up a tasty meal.

Can you eat things that aren't on this list? Sure! Just don't do it *too* often, especially when you're starting out. Have one treat meal a week—not a cheat meal, because you're *treating* yourself—and you'll do great.

If you're still finding it difficult to eat healthy, there's something that can help: meal prepping.

COOK A LOT, SAVE A LOT, EAT HEALTHIER

Like many humans, I eat out more than I should. Especially in weeks when my job's gotten busy or I've felt like things are getting out of control, I know I can always grab some fast food—even if it's from a healthier place—and it makes me feel like I'm more in control and using my time better.

But that's kind of a problem, especially when I'm trying to save money, stay in shape, and save time. Instead, what I try to do more often than not, even during busy weeks, is prepare my meals in advance.

If you struggle at all with your eating, you should meal-prep. If you have loved ones you need to cook for on a regular basis—and you're all trying to eat healthier—you should meal-prep.

It takes one of the hardest parts of maintaining a healthy diet—deciding what to eat—and makes it easier.

Before I give you some tips on how to do it, here's why you should try it:

1. **It saves time.** One of the main reasons I hate making my own meals is because it takes so long. Even if it's only twenty minutes to prepare and cook your food for each meal, that's an hour a day. But if you spend one hour cooking all your meals for the week, you've saved almost six hours of cooking.

2. **It saves money.** Instead of spending $8 to $10 per meal by eating out (and that's cheap), if you buy your food in bulk, you can end up making each meal cost only $2 to $3, depending on the quality of ingredients you use. So instead of spending potentially $24 a day on meals, you're now spending $6, or saving about $100 a week. That's enough money to buy at least five copies of this book a week, which, studies have proved, will make my publisher much happier.

3. **It keeps you on track.** You know what your meals are going to be if you've already planned them out in advance. If you don't have anything to eat or haven't planned out your meals, you're more likely to make some bad decisions. This helps keep your options limited and makes it easier for you to stick to better choices.

4. **It's easier to track your meals.** If you've portioned everything in advance, you more or less know how much food you're eating. That means if you aren't seeing the results you want, you know you can adjust your food intake accordingly.

5. **It's stress relieving.** I've never, ever been someone who likes to cook. But something about cooking a ton of food all at once and storing it for the rest of the week is so relaxing. I put on a podcast, make a ton of food, and feel like I'm some failed Parisian chef who somehow developed a Midwestern accent. It feels good when you're done. Not to mention, you're setting yourself up for a higher chance of success that week, which can make you feel less stressed overall. For me, watching YouTube videos of people doing meal prep is like a vacation.

Now that I've convinced you with my sweet list, here's how you do it.

PICK YOUR MEAL(S)

When you're making all your meals for the week, you've got to get used to eating more or less the same thing every day. Here's an example of a meal you can make a ton of just by cooking a few main ingredients:

- Chicken
- Broccoli
- Brown rice

This is the bodybuilder's special. There are thousands of people with fantastic biceps and skinny waists who eat a few meals a day made with just these ingredients. You can add pepper, salt, barbecue sauce, coconut oil, or whatever you like to make it a bit more flavorful, and so you get some more of those much-needed fats. But overall, these three ingredients are easy to make, even for a dummy like me.

You don't have to make a meal with exactly those ingredients, but it gives you a general idea to focus on a few main things that you can cook more or less the same way: a healthy protein, veggies, and some fats. Nuts, such as almonds, are a great source of fat. So is cheese. (I have definitely made cheese sticks a regular part of my meal-prep plan.)

Pick something that you know you can make. And if you're scared of the kitchen, like I still somewhat am, you can easily find great cooking resources on YouTube. Or you can call my mom and she'll set you straight.

Get your ingredients

Figure out how many ingredients you need for a single meal, then multiply that by the number of meals you plan on having that week.

For instance, if you're going to eat two of these meals a day—maybe one for lunch and one for dinner, which means you can still have the same breakfast as your family or try to spice things up in the morning—you would need enough ingredients to make fourteen meals.

You'll probably also need some containers, preferably micro-wavable, to store all your meals in. It's much easier to make each meal its own separate thing, instead of keeping the final parts of the meals in their own separate containers. It's much less work for you when it comes to chowtime.

Find a day when you can get your shopping and cooking done. Make a list. Head to the grocery store and get what you need. Next comes the most fun part.

Cook it all at once

Put on your chef's apron (and preferably giant chef's hat) and get ready to make some food. If you're a more experienced cook, you can do multiple things at once, such as cut up your meat while your veg-gies are cooking. If you're like me, you can still do things one at a time and it'll be all good.

Finish each of your ingredients and portion them into each meal container. If you're really set on counting calories, this is when you can weigh things to make sure they're all equal. (Or, for some foods, like beef or turkey patties, you can weigh them before you cook them to make sure they're all even.)

I would suggest trying to make some sort of sauce you can put over your meat, like barbecue, so when you reheat the food later it'll help keep it not only flavorful but also a little less dry.

Depending on how many meals you're going to eat in a day, I would suggest putting the next four or five days' worth of meals in the fridge and the rest in the freezer. That way they'll stay fresh and tasty. (I am told that leftovers, as long as fish isn't involved, can usually last up to ten days in the fridge. Use the smell test to decide if something's still good.)

Cooking all your week's meals in advance isn't for everyone. But for those who are already thinking to themselves that this sounds boring, that they would get tired of eating the same thing over and over again, I'll point this out: Eating a wide variety of meals all the time is definitely what got me to my unhealthiest point.

Also, almost every nation in the world has some way to cook chicken and they're all different. Spices and sauces are magic.

While variety can be good, if you're in a place you don't want to be when it comes to your body, try eating boring for a while. Depending on how good your cooking skills are, you can probably make tasty *and* healthy food, and cook a few different options during your weekly meal prep, so you're not eating the exact same thing every day.

Or, if you're more adventurous, take a Sunday to make several different meals that you can pack in your freezer—these extra options can last you a few weeks and give you more variety.

EAT A LITTLE LESS, NOT A LOT LESS

We've talked about this before—your body burns calories to make fuel. If it has those calories coming in the form of food, cool; it digests that and uses it. If it doesn't have enough, it needs to find it elsewhere on your body, through fat and muscle.

For most people, what they want to lose is the fat, but maintain the muscle.

Our bodies are constantly acting out of fear that we may never eat again. So if you suddenly stop eating entirely, your body freaks out and starts to go through some rapid changes, many of which are meant to compel you to start eating a lot.

This is why if you're trying to lose weight, you need to do it slowly. Because if you do it fast, you're not going to have a great time.

Let's say your goal is to lose twenty-five pounds. If you lost twenty-five pounds in a month, that'd be bad. It'd mean you were losing about five pounds a week. Or maybe you just chopped off one of your legs. (Don't do this.)

Here are some potential side effects of starving yourself like this:

- Hair loss
- Lack of sex drive
- Muscle loss
- Increased irritability
- Higher chance of gaining back the weight you lost

It's not good to starve yourself in an attempt to lose weight. It shouldn't be completely awful and terrible to try to get yourself to a different weight. Because if it sucks, you'll stop trying. And if the diet is excruciating to maintain, why would you want to keep doing that? Life should be fun, dammit.

(As I've mentioned, I've been able to lose twenty pounds in a month through extreme diet and exercise. Did I gain it all back and then some? Yup! The only weight I've managed to keep off for multiple years is the seventy or so pounds I lost slowly over the course of more than a year. Everything after that, where I went too fast, I gained back.)

Life shouldn't constantly suck. Neither should changing your lifestyle to meet your health and fitness goals. So instead, here's what you need to do:

LOSE WEIGHT SLOWLY

One pound a week. That's all you need to lose. More than that really isn't necessary, unless you're severely overweight. (And if that's the case, you should be talking to your doctor instead of relying on books written by people like me.)

Let's say you've stayed around the same weight for some time, perhaps two hundred pounds. You maybe go up a pound or two, but you kind of hover around this area. That means you're probably eating enough to sustain your weight, or what some would call *caloric maintenance*. What you're looking to do is go into a *caloric deficit*, or eating enough so your body has to find its calories elsewhere.

One pound a week is attainable for most people. One pound is equal to 3,500 calories. Even though I don't think counting calories is the perfect way to lose weight, all you need to do is eat 500 fewer calories a day, or work out enough to burn 500 calories, or a mix of both.

Here's an example of how to do this: Let's say you regularly eat one delicious candy bar a day. The last time I checked, those averaged about 250 calories. And if you're, say, a two-hundred-pound person, if you walk at a normal pace, you'll lose about 100 calories per mile. So if you just don't have that candy bar and walk 2.5 miles a day, poof, that'll get you to those 500 calories a day.

Let's check our math: That's 500 calories a day, times seven days, which comes to 3,500 calories. That's one pound. And it's not *that much* extra work. You don't need to go to the gym and lift a ton of weights. You don't have to stop eating all your favorite meals. As long as you were already maintaining your existing weight, this should help you get where you want to go.

It's not going to happen overnight. But you didn't gain all the weight overnight, either. It was put on gradually, over many years. That means if you lose one pound a week, after about five or six months, that'll average out to twenty-five pounds.

What if I continue to gain weight?

Unless that's your goal (and yes, there are people who try to gain weight on purpose, and that's also quite okay!), then you need to figure out how many calories you *should* be eating a day to maintain your weight. This can be a little hard, and it's by no means perfect, but what you should do is spend a week writing down everything you eat regularly.

Don't overthink it; just keep track of it all. Most of us eat the same handful of meals regularly, or go to the same places for lunch, or have a similar routine when it comes to meals.

At the end of the seven days, weigh yourself. Then find a website to calculate your TDEE, or total daily energy expenditure. (Just google for one; they're all pretty much the same.) This will show you how many calories you need just to survive, or what your body burns just by existing. If you don't move a lot in your job, or if you're not physically active, you'll need fewer than someone who does. (Which is okay!)

Next, using the list of food you ate during the last week, figure out the calories in everything you ate. See how many calories you ate in a day, on average. Is it more than how much you need a day? If you've been gaining weight, it probably is. If you still think you're eating *fewer* calories than your body needs, a few things could have happened:

1. You didn't include all the food you ate. Did you remember your snacks? That cookie you had from the break room? The double seven-shot, no-foam, two-pumps-of-cinnamon latte? All these add up, so include them.
2. You calculated your calories incorrectly because math is hard.
3. You made much larger portions than you thought, because you either didn't count or weigh the ingredients you were us-

ing. (Weighing your food, you may be asking? Yup. How else
will you know your true portion sizes in relation to their supposed calorie counts?)

4. The food labels were incorrect on how many calories were in
the food.

5. You could actually have an underlying medical problem and
should see a doctor to check it out. (This is much, much rarer
than you think.)

What you should try to do is cut back on what you're eating and
give it another week. What you're attempting to do is a little science
experiment about yourself, getting some data to help you come up
with a hypothesis.

What's the hypothesis? You're eating more calories than your
body needs. Once you have the data showing this to be the case, you
can start to make changes. That muffin you have every morning?
It's 500 calories! Do you really need that? Maybe not. How about that
bag of chips you have after your 3:00 p.m. daily meeting? It's 350 calories.

All these things add up. And what you need to do is figure out
what you can eliminate to get you to the number of calories you need
to maintain your weight. That's your first goal.

Once you get there, next, see the previous section and start cutting just 250 to 500 calories a day, either by eating less or moving
more, or both.

And just in case I haven't made this clear enough: Your weight
isn't the be-all, end-all describer of your health and fitness. That's
more of a personal thing, or something between you and medical
professionals.

Is your blood pressure okay? Does your blood work come back as
okay? Cool—you're probably pretty healthy!

Can you do the activities you want that bring you joy? Great! Do you have a good-enough amount of energy to get through the day? Wonderful.

If you want to fix aesthetic things, that's just a battle between your percentage of muscle mass and body fat, keeping the former larger and the latter smaller. But otherwise, focusing on the other parts of your life as a sign of good health and fitness? All good things.

■ ■ ■

Sounds easy, huh? It is on paper. But trust me, it can be hard for many, especially when starting out. I know it was for me. If you need further help, refer back to chapter 8 for some good tips on pushing yourself toward better decisions.

I THINK YOU SHOULD LIFT WEIGHTS

Strength training, or lifting weights, should be a part of your regular routine if you're trying to get healthier.

When I say "lifting weights," I mean lifting either a barbell or a dumbbell, or using resistance bands or something that causes you to push your major muscle groups toward exhaustion through repeated motions. That can be accomplished in a lot of different ways. But it usually requires equipment.

Note: *Bodyweight calisthenics, where you use your own body and do push-ups or sit-ups or whatever, is a good start, or can complement a strength-training routine. (This includes yoga.) But in general, I think you should be moving some weight around.*

Here's why you should lift weights:

1. It helps you maintain your muscles.

If you consume fewer calories than your body needs, you'll lose weight. But unless you're actively working your muscles, you'll lose muscle as well as fat. And if you're going for a look that's generally considered more pleasing to folks, maintaining that muscle tone is important. Doing strength training just a few days a week will help you maintain the muscles you already have while losing some of the fat.

2. It helps you **_build_** muscle.

Some people are able to lose fat and gain muscle at the same time. Not everyone, of course. But the best way to do this is through strength training. If you have more muscles on your body, you'll look, at least in the Western world, a bit more aesthetically pleasing. It'll help your body look leaner when you have more muscles. Your clothes will fit better, too!

3. More muscle means more calories burned.

If you have more muscles, your body will burn more calories while you just exist. So by maintaining, or building, muscle mass, you'll be able to lose weight faster than you would with less muscle mass.

4. Exercise burns calories.

When you lift weights, you do burn some calories. Maybe not as many as in traditional cardio, but you'll definitely have burned off some energy.

5. You burn more calories **_after_** exercising.

This one is kind of nuts: In the hours after lifting weights, your body burns more calories at rest than it had prior to exercising, in a process referred to as "excess post-exercise oxygen consumption."[1] It's like you get all these added benefits, as if you were working out longer and harder than you really are. By lifting weights, you set yourself up for even more weight-loss success.

6. It helps you lead an active life.

Not everyone wants to do Tough Mudders and climb walls and run ten miles for "fun" on the weekend. But you probably want to be able to throw a Frisbee with your friends, chase after your kids, or dance the night away at a wedding. The more strength you have (as well as aerobic conditioning!), the more you're able to do these things and stay active at any age.

7. It'll help you in old age.

Starting at age fifty, those who don't do any strength training can begin to lose about 1 percent of their muscle mass a year, and that amount increases as you age.[2] This is why some people get into their seventies and are no longer strong enough to put on clothing, or walk upright, or do many everyday activities. Strength training helps you build and maintain that muscle mass before you get old, and can even do the same when you get to those ages. (Although, of course, you can't stop *all* muscle mass loss as you age, you can slow it down a bit.) Weight lifting isn't only for the old. Anyone can do it. So you should, as you're anyone.

8. It helps your heart.

Lifting weights has cardiovascular benefits, too. Even though strength training is quite different from cardio, your body needs oxygen and fast-moving blood when you decide to lift something heavy. This means that as your muscles get stronger, so do the parts of your body that power those muscles.

9. It's pretty cool to learn what your body can do.

The first time I was able to squat my body weight, I cried. I never knew my body was capable of lifting 250 pounds, hanging on a barbell, on my back. And yet there I was, racking that sucker off the squat rack, dropping down, and popping back up. It was amazing to discover that, in just a few months, I was able to make my body strong enough to throw the equivalent of *me* on my back and move it. If you include my own body weight, that meant I was moving almost *a quarter of a ton*. That's what you discover when lifting weights—you can accomplish more than you ever thought possible, much faster than you thought it'd ever be.

10. It gives you purpose.

You will quickly discover lifting weights becomes slightly addictive. Not because you're all "MORE WEIGHT" like some accused Salem witch-trial participant. But because it gives you a goal to accomplish on a regular basis. You wake up knowing you're going to head to the gym later and attempt to do something your body hasn't done before—lift more weight than you did previously. You're always attempting to level up. So if you don't have a lot going for you, lifting weights can give you something to kick ass at. And it feels great.

11. It can be done in addition to cardio.

If you don't wanna make lifting weights the only thing you do, that's fine! You don't *have* to lift weights. Some folks may just want to lose a few pounds, and cardio *definitely* can help you with that—if you burn more calories than your body needs, you lose weight. What lifting weights definitely helps out with is aesthetics: It helps you gain better proportions, which can actually help *hide* your belly fat, because now you've got wider shoulders for men; and for women, it can help you increase the curves you want. If you do only cardio, and if you're already pear-shaped, you may just remain pear-shaped, albeit a smaller pear. And that's fine! But just know that if you're able to maintain more of your muscle mass while losing weight, you won't get suddenly bigger and bulky. You'll instead have clothes that fit better.

■ ■ ■

Not everyone is physically capable of lifting weights, for a wide variety of reasons. But I've seen people in wheelchairs benching more than I ever could. I've seen people missing limbs who use prosthetics and do more pull-ups than I can imagine. You may also have your own issues that prevent you from lifting properly, or safely. So always check with a doctor to make sure you're physically capable.

But I think everyone can benefit from more strength training. Go try it a few times a week and make it a part of your regular routine. Search for a beginner program online and then stick to it for twelve weeks before you tweak it. (Get rid of the idea that there's a perfect routine: Unless you're trying to be a bodybuilder or professional athlete, you can choose any full-body routine, including one I've included on the next page.)

Your body will love you for it.

Note: The U.S. Department of Health and Human Services suggests you should strength-train at least twice a week, hitting all the major muscle groups at a moderate intensity or more. (It also suggests at least 150 to 300 minutes of moderate-intensity aerobic activity, or 75 to 150 minutes of vigorous-intensity aerobic activity. See? Cardio's not all bad!)[3]

This shows you don't need to Hulk-out and work toward being an Adonis or Aphrodite. (Unless, of course, you want to be.) One hour a day, including warming up your muscles, three times a week is more than enough for most people. For once, you can trust the government.

BASIC STRENGTH-TRAINING WORKOUT

This is set up to be a three-day-a-week, full-body workout, which you can do if you have access to dumbbells and a bench, as well as other basic equipment, with one day of rest in between.

Note: If you wanna also do cardio, sure! If you wanna add some ab stuff at the end (if you have time), sure! I've included suggestions for that.

"But, Andy, what weight do I start at?"

Start with the lowest you have! Work your way up until you can do 12 reps with good form and you begin to slow down, where it finally starts to feel *hard*. If you can do a bench press with 15-pound dumbbells in each hand for 12 reps, next try 20 pounds. If that goes swell, then try 25. If you can only do 8 to 10 reps of 25, bingo—you've found your starting weight.

The idea is to find a weight you can do between 8 to 12 reps for three sets. Once you can do 12 reps for three sets during your regular planned workout, it's time to up the weight to the next amount! And so on and so on and so on until you are mega-strong.

Let's dive into your workout. You'll have Workout A, which focuses on quads, chest, midback, and biceps; and Workout B, which focuses on hamstrings/glutes, shoulders, upper back, and triceps. The idea is to switch between each, going every other workout. Your schedule would thus look like this:

Week One:

Monday: Workout A
Wednesday: Workout B
Friday: Workout A

Week Two:

Monday: Workout B
Wednesday: Workout A
Friday: Workout B

And so on and so on.

An important note: *Program hopping is a thing lots of people do, especially when they're a beginner at strength training. Whether you choose this exercise plan or another, stick with it for three months before deciding you want to try some other strength-training plan. That's about how long it'll take before you start to see changes in your body, even though many see changes sooner. You'll get more motivation after you see your body begin to change, which means you're more likely to keep working out.*

Here are the workouts. All exercises are 3 sets of 8 to 12 reps, unless otherwise noted.

Workout A:

Leg press
Hamstring curl machine
Dumbbell bench/machine bench
One-arm dumbbell row
Bicep curl (This can be totally a low-ass weight and that's just fine! Also, switch between traditional and hammer curls on every other workout.)
Side planks (optional, mostly if you hate yourself)—3x30 seconds on each side

Workout B:

Dumbell single-leg squat
Hamstring curl machine

Sitting dumbbell shoulder press/machine overhead press
Lat pull-down
Dumbell tricep extension (behind the head, and again, it can
    be a totally low weight)
Front planks (optional, mostly if you hate yourself)—
    3x30 seconds

For the first three lifts on each workout, rest between 60 and 120 seconds between each set, depending on how easy the set was. For the final three, rest only 60 seconds.

At the beginning of your first two or three lifts, be sure to warm up. Don't immediately start with what we call your "working sets," or the sets that are part of that day's workout.

Instead, begin by doing one set of 12 at half the weight, then another set around 75 percent of the weight, then another at 85 to 90 percent. Take short breaks between each, and feel free to decrease the amount of reps as the weight goes up so you don't tire yourself out before your actual sets. This will help warm your muscles up and get your blood flowing, which is important in preventing injuries, and also in getting you primed to be as strong as possible during your lifts.

As soon as you're able to do three sets of 12 reps at a certain weight, and maintain good form, go up to the next weight.

GENERAL EXERCISE ADVICE

Your exercise regimen should be so easy it can fit on a Post-it Note, especially if you're just starting out. Anything more complicated than that and you're setting yourself up for failure.

Save the hard work for your muscles, not your brain.

Now, I haven't given you complete explanations of how to do each exercise movement for a reason. That's because you're going to find much better instructions from the videos on YouTube showing you how to do each exercise than if I took photos showing each or used words to describe the actions. That's how I learned the basic movements—and sometimes I would take videos and share them with my friends who lifted weights and they'd give me pointers.

What if your gym doesn't have any of these weights or machines? Google to find alternatives. And while I had a whole chapter about using barbells in your workouts, I think dumbbells are a lot easier and less scary for newbies.

This routine is more about building a habit. It's similar to the one that got me started on my fitness journey, so I thought maybe it'd help you, too. (Not to mention, it's the basic one I wrote up for my girlfriend at the time, and it worked out quite well for her.)

It's not a perfect workout plan—and that's the point. None of them are. I am sure others will gladly email to tell me how it's wrong or bad, but guess what? If it gets you motivated and going to the gym, then it's doing its job.

That's the basic workout plan. Go forth and seek swollness!

LOOSE SKIN

If you gain a lot of weight, especially if you've carried it for years, your body deals with it by stretching your skin. This is why people get stretch marks.

Here's the truth: Everyone gets stretch marks. Even body-builders, because they, too, are increasing their body mass and causing their skin to stretch. Stretch marks are normal. Everyone has them.

That means if you lose a good deal of weight, there's a chance your skin may not snap back completely, and you'll have some loose skin. This will depend on how old you are, how much weight you gained, and how much you lost. Some people may have a little loose skin; some may have a lot. It's just something that happens.

If you lost your weight superfast, you're more likely to have loose skin than if you lost it slowly. (Another reason you should take your time with weight loss.) And if you retain muscle mass, that will also help out, because it gives you something to fill the space. (Another reason to lift weights.) Other than that, there's not a lot you can do, outside of surgery.

For some people, the skin is a bit more elastic, and it will move back. Others will still have a bit of loose skin. But it's natural. One thing you can do is try to build more muscle after you've hit a goal weight. It's a slow process, but that's one option.

Otherwise, you can just live with your loose skin like the rest of us. Nobody who's ever seen me shirtless (hellooooooooo, lucky people!) has ever brought up how my tummy has a bit of loose skin. If they ever thought negatively about it, they haven't said it. At least to my face. I notice it, but nobody else seems to—even my girlfriend at the time didn't know what I was talking about when I asked her about it. We all may notice our own faults more than others do, so it may not even be something others notice about you.

If someone thinks you're gross because you have some loose skin, that person is an asshole and their opinion doesn't matter. And you don't need them in your life anyway.

Loose skin is something you should be proud of, not ashamed of. It means you worked hard to get in better shape. Or you had a baby! (Probably less likely to happen for cis men.) And regardless of how you lived your life, everyone's skin eventually loses its elasticity and gets a bit loose. That's just natural. So is what's happened to you.

Some people don't want to lose weight because they're afraid of having excess skin. But here's the deal: Losing weight will help you with all sorts of other health-related maladies. It'll also help with so many other things, like making your clothes fit better, boosting your confidence, and much more. The benefits of losing weight definitely outweigh the cons of loose skin. Trust me on this.

Depending on the skin amount, there are surgeries available. They come with their own issues, of course, and you should discuss them with your doctor. In many instances, they won't let you do the surgery until you've managed to keep the weight off for years, which I think is a good thing.

In the meantime, wear that loose skin with pride. It's a badge of honor. And I think it makes you look awesome.

WALK MORE

Running isn't for everyone. Neither is lifting weights. Or going to a Pilates class. Or whatever else exists out there that makes you sweat a lot. Even though I like certain activities, or your friends do, doesn't mean you will.

But there *is* one thing that most of us can do that is supereffective at weight loss and a great low-impact exercise: walking.

You may be like, "Oh, that thing I do every day to get from my house to my car in the driveway?" Yes, that thing. Where you move one leg and then the other in a slow manner, usually not causing you to breathe heavy or sweat a lot. Walking.

Here are some of the many reasons it's a great form of exercise:

1. **You can do it almost anywhere.** Most cities have sidewalks, or at least roads you can walk on the side of. Some even have nice parks. Or pretty downtown areas. You just put one foot in front of the other and go.

2. **It isn't too strenuous.** I know some people have issues walking, but for the rest of us, it's something we've been doing since we were toddlers. (That and drawing on walls with crayons. Wait, you don't still do that?) Most of us can walk a mile with no problems.

3. **It actually burns a lot of calories.** Even though you aren't exerting yourself too much, walking still increases the number of calories you burn. It may be a *bit* fewer than burned while running, but actually not by much. A two-hundred-pound person would burn about 150 calories running one mile in ten minutes. That same person walking one mile in twenty minutes? About 120 calories.

4. **It's easier on your body.** Lifting weights and running and other forms of exercise can be a bit tough on your joints. Walking, however, is not as bad. It still gets your blood flowing, and it can elevate your heart rate, so you still get some of those added benefits, too.

5. **You can listen to great books.** During my walks, I listen to audiobooks and podcasts. So not only am I getting healthier, but I'm also getting entertained and smarter at the same time. Working out my body *and* my brain? Win-win!

6. **It's a great way to start getting in the exercise habit.** Setting up a goal every day for a certain amount of time or number of steps to walk is, I think, much easier than getting into the habit of doing other forms of exercise. You can walk on your lunch break, or during a business call, or while taking your pet outside. It's much harder to do a full-body workout while on a business call, let me tell you.

True story: I heard about my first book deal while at the gym and pretended like I could pay attention while doing curls. (I could not, and my agent made me take a break from weight lifting. One of his many good ideas.)

Now that I've proved walking is clearly something you should be doing regularly, let's talk about what you should look for when you decide to take up walking:

1. **Shoot for a goal.** It can be as simple as walking 10,000 steps a day. Or if you need some time to work up to that, you can start at 5,000 steps. Don't like steps? How about if you go for two 30-minute walks a day? Or twice around the block? Whatever it is, make a goal and then do it every day.

2. **Track your progress.** Most smartphones come with some method of tracking your steps. While they're not the most accurate—neither are those expensive pedometers—they are at least something most of us have around a lot of the time. So you can be absentmindedly hitting your walking goals just with your daily activities!

3. **Push yourself.** Let's say you've set a goal of 10,000 steps a day. For the past two weeks, you've been hitting it every day, and then some. Next you should increase it, let's say to 12,000 steps a day. After you've comfortably hit that goal, increase it again. And so on, and so on. There was a time where I was regularly walking 20,000 steps a day. (Yes, I listened to *a lot* of audiobooks.) Depending on how much cardio I'm doing, I at least hit 10,000, but these days some of that is through running.

4. **Set your day up to walk more.** I work from home, so sometimes instead of making my meals in my kitchen, and because

I can afford to do so, I tend to go for a walk to somewhere in my neighborhood for food. Most of the best spots are at least half a mile away. If all I do is walk there and back, that's about a mile of my daily goal. Same thing for most dinners, too. But I usually like to walk during my entire lunch break, down quiet streets, checking shops in my area, saying hi to friends. You probably have regular events in your life where you can add in a few extra steps, too. Got a meeting and it's two miles away, but you'd normally drive and the weather's nice? Leave earlier and go for a walk. Have some writing to do? Walk to a nearby park and do it on a bench. You can always find more ways to push yourself to walk more.

5. **Find new places to walk.** If you're regularly taking hour-long walks some days, you'll discover your regular walking areas can tend to get boring. I live in Chicago, where if you walk two miles in one direction, you're usually in an entirely different neighborhood, so I'm a bit lucky. Sometimes I'll take a train or bus somewhere and then walk the distance back. When I'm visiting other cities, I like to drive to parts of town that are nice (and safe; always a good thing to check) and then walk around for a few hours.

6. **You don't *only* have to walk.** I run a few days most weeks, more if I'm training for a race. I'm more concerned about total steps than how fast I took them. If you like to walk *and* run, that's great! You can do both. Don't feel like you have to only do one or the other.

I got my parents into walking more a few years ago. The first few weeks were hard for them, as they tried to go a mile in one walk around their neighborhood. But now they can regularly walk a few miles without issue. Their bodies adapted, helped them get stronger and get used to longer walks. They're healthier because of it. And you can do the same.

Also: The FDA suggests you should do 150 minutes a week of moderate cardio. That's potentially 30 minutes a day of walking five times a week.

FIDO AS YOUR WORKOUT PARTNER

Want another way to force yourself to walk more? It's simple: Get a dog.

A good friend of mine gave me this advice. If you have a dog, and if you aren't a crappy owner, you have to take the dog outside for walks. Therefore, you have to go outside for walks. While it's a big commitment to bring a pet into your world, if you can't find other reasons to make you get out and move, getting an animal who loves you may just do it.

EXCUSEITIS, OR HOW NOT TO FIND THE TIME

I used to suffer from a debilitating illness that affects billions of people. Sometimes I still suffer from it, because there is no known cure. But I have a lot of great ways to battle it so it has less control over my body.

Yes, I am talking about excuseitis.

Excuseitis is the disease many of us have that says we have reasons we can't get healthier. One of the biggest symptoms of excuseitis is saying you don't have enough time, or energy, or willpower to achieve your fitness goals.

I hear it a lot from people who are incredibly intelligent, successful professionals who have so much going for them. But then they say, because of their career, or their hobbies, or maybe even their family, they don't have time to eat healthy, to exercise, or to give a damn about their bodies.

Those are all excuses.

And I'm the king of excuses.

Every time I order a pizza and eat all of it, I tell myself I was too busy to make food, so it was fine for me to eat unhealthily. (Guess what I do while eating the pizza? Watch TV and lounge around.)

Every time I skip the gym because I'm super busy and have lots of other plans, I usually end up staying home and doing nothing.

An excuse is just another opportunity for you to deny yourself the chance of achieving your goals. Whenever I tell myself another excuse for why I can't do something I've planned out, first I forgive myself. Then I try to take one tiny step toward whatever I'm attempting to excuse my way out of.

It could be I wanted to skip the gym. So I'll put on my exercise outfit and sit on the couch. Baby steps. And then I'll get annoyed that I am on the couch in running shorts and I'll go exercise.

Or maybe I don't want to make myself dinner and want to order in and eat five times the number of calories I need. I'll go to the stove, put a pan on it, and turn on the flame. Well, I'm practically cooking now—might as well finish it.

You can always find excuses

You can make every excuse possible for why you fall back into your old behaviors. It's totally natural. I remember one time walking to the gym, my headphones blaring music, and I suddenly decided I didn't want to go, with my whole body screaming that I was a failure, that I shouldn't even try to lift weights because I was just a mess. Then, just as I was about to get back to my apartment building, my phone's random playlist decided to play Simon and Garfunkel's "Bridge Over Troubled Water."

Because sometimes the universe is funny.

I started to cry, mostly because the song starts off about feeling tired and like you don't matter, and also because the bridge is incredibly uplifting. It made me feel like even though right now I felt shitty, I could still do this. I turned around and lifted a bunch of weight and it was fine.

Bet you didn't expect someone to ever tell you how Simon and Garfunkel helped them to go squat a few hundred pounds, but now you have.

Find your own 1970s piano falsetto ballad that pushes you out of your own existential funk and back into your good habits. You'll never cure your excuseitis, but you can make it less powerful and manage it.

Personal responsibility is exactly that: personal. And you're responsible for it. While many things are in fact out of your control, what you do with your time is something you can have more of a handle on.

How to find the time

We are all busy, or so we all say, which is just another part of excuseitis. And with all the additions of modern technology invading our every waking moment in the last decade, it *feels* like we're busier than ever.

Some studies back this up, to a degree. But other studies show we are actually working *less* in America than we used to, and that our leisure time is up, especially if you're less educated.[4]

When I was researching and writing this book, I worked a full-time job, managing a half-dozen employees, all while regularly exercising, traveling to give talks, writing, and teaching. My friends always asked how the hell I was capable of doing it all.

Because I made time for it. And I continue to make time.

Usually, when friends ask for help with their fitness goals, they're looking for a better way to eat or information on how to lift weights or train for a race. And then they say the same thing over and over whenever I give them suggestions: "But I don't have time for all that!"

I'll give them some ways of finding the time, and they'll shake their heads. "I just don't have the time. What else can I do?"

Not making time for our health is how a lot of us got to where we are to begin with. Throughout my twenties, I had a ton of free time, even with a full-time job. How did I spend it? Watching television, hanging out at bars, eating fast food. But when it came to my health and fitness? Didn't have time to do anything about *that*.

I was busy sitting at a bar or fast-food place reading a book! Soooooooo busy.

Now that I'm in my early thirties, I'm busier than ever. My days are jam-packed with my full-time job, events after work, classes I take, classes I teach, and, well, these book things I like to write. Yet I can still find time to work out regularly and eat not *too* badly most of the time.

Here's how to do it:

- **Schedule your life.** My calendar shows all my appointments, work meetings, date nights, everything I need to keep track of. On top of that, I'll put my planned workouts into my calendar.

- **Count your time.** If you don't think you have enough time, spend a week writing down everything you do before and after work. You may think you don't have a lot of time, but how much of your day is spent waiting in line at a coffee shop or at a restaurant on your lunch break? Probably just as much time as it would've taken to make that coffee or food yourself.

- **Watch less television.** This is one of the hardest ones. We as a species love to sit and watch our stories. It's relaxing. It's wonderful. But you can accomplish an entire workout, or go for a run or a good walk, during the time it takes to watch two episodes of *The Office*.

- **Tell your family you need the time.** I know for those who have families, it's much harder to eat healthy and find time to work out. For some, that may mean asking your significant other or another family member to give you an hour every few days to go exercise. (And you, obviously, can do the same for them.) Many of my friends with kids get up extra early to work out before their little ones wake up. You can also schedule family outings that involve walking, or running, or something that gets you moving. When I visit my parents, we regularly go on walks and chat.

- **Tell your employer you need the time.** This is hard for some people to do, and it depends on the type of job you have, but a healthy person is a more productive person. You can make the case to your boss that you need to head out to exercise in the early afternoon, or to make a grocery-shopping run, so you can stay healthy. Of course, you may need to stay an hour later, but at least ask if you're able to do this. For those with salaried jobs, this is definitely easier, but not everyone has this luxury.

- **Prep your meals.** Instead of spending the time making meals every day, make them all one day a week. You don't have to make every single meal the same when you do this, either—you can make a variety, so your diet varies. Even if you have a family you need to cook for, this can save a lot of time and give you some flexibility when it comes to what to cook. (Check out the earlier section on meal prepping.)

- **Do less stuff.** One thing I've realized as I get older is that I'm often spread thinner than I would like. I've cut out some things from my life that either weren't as rewarding or I just knew I wouldn't have the time to devote to. Case in point: In late 2017, I started taking piano lessons again. (It's been about twenty years.) But I quickly realized, because of a large work project that was taking up a lot of my free time, I could either practice every day for an hour or exercise. Getting better at playing the piano wasn't as important to me, in the long term, as being healthier, so I decided to cancel my piano lessons. You may have to do the same in your own life. (It's true: You can't have it all.)

Finding time can be frustrating. **But you need to make the time for your health, or else it just won't happen.** I am the king of excuses when it comes to my health, because, as I've already told you, I suffer from excuseitis. You can find any reason for *why* you *can't* make the effort. If you think hard enough, I also believe you can then discover reasons about why you *can* make the effort, too.

PERFECTION ISN'T REAL

And finally, one of the big brain hurdles we all have to get over is this idea of perfection. It's one of the most important points in figuring out how to make this all work for you.

Perfection with our bodies, with our work, with our art. Because here's the truth: Perfection isn't actually attainable in anything. You can only push yourself closer to what someone—maybe you, dear reader?—has *decided* is perfection.

That's in anything—nobody can play a Mozart sonata perfectly. Nobody has a perfect body. Nobody's car is perfect. (My dad and his Corvette would beg to differ, I'm sure.)

But media has planted this insidious virus inside us that we are *absolute failures* if we're not perfect at whatever we do. If you try to pick up the guitar and aren't immediately Jimi Hendrix, you're a failure. If you can't immediately run a marathon the first time you put on a pair of shoes, failure. If you spend one week eating healthy and your body doesn't look like someone's on a magazine cover, failure.

Total crap.

You see only success in our popular media—especially social media. You don't see failures and mistakes. You don't see someone practicing guitar twelve hours a day so they can play a riff perfectly.

You don't see 5:00 a.m. runs for six months before someone does a marathon. You don't see the meals eaten, the calories tracked, the cooking someone does to look great on a magazine cover, not to mention the years of exercise *plus* probably some really great genes. (And, depending on the magazine in question, probably a *bunch* of airbrushing.)

You have to beat this into your mind right now: Nothing is perfect. Most of all, not your body. We're all so unique, so different, that even if we had a rubric for how to decide what makes a body perfect, nobody would possibly be able to match it.

Like, I don't even have two legs that are the same length. One of my ears is way higher on my head than the other. The hair on the top of my head has decided to retire early. I'm not perfect.

But I'm pretty damn good. And so are you.

Of course we can push ourselves to be better. To look better. To perform better. But don't ever feel bad that you're not *perfect*. Be happy that you're you, and that you're trying.

Because if you're trying, you're already succeeding.

FINAL TAKEAWAYS

For more than a year and a half, I spent almost all my free time researching fitness, attempting to get in better shape, and caring more about my body—and my mind—than I ever have before. Especially during grueling workouts, or when I was eating the same meal for the fifth or sixth time that week, I wondered whether this was worth it.

Life seemed so much simpler when I was in worse shape. I *seemed* to have more free time. I did whatever I wanted. I ate whatever—and whenever—I wanted. My body had fewer aches and pains. I had a million percent less sweaty shirts and shorts that needed washing every week.

It seemed as though my life was better before all of this.

It wasn't.

When I think back on my older life, I used to be sick constantly. I hated looking at myself in the mirror. I hadn't accomplished anything athletic.

I was a nerdy, brainy kid. I always thought exercise and caring about your health and fitness was for *other* people, not people like me who liked movies and books and musicals. (Because wow, Andy, *nobody* likes those things. You're so unique!)

But all this has definitely been worth it.

Growing up, I was more interested in reading Stephen King novels and listening to obscure punk bands than trying out for the track team. For many of my friends, being active was just part of their life. It never was for me. I never truly knew the joy—and also the heartache—that can come when you attempt to push your body, and your mind, further than you thought possible.

Now I know all that and more.

Because of the research for this book, I've run two half marathons, which, technically, *technically*, means I've run a full marathon. (All the people who have actually run marathons are screaming at me while reading this.) I've tested my cardiovascular ability through scientific means, and I am above the "superior" level for someone my age. I've taken my body from a relatively unhealthy amount of body fat (30 percent) and gotten it to a healthier level (25 percent). I've also managed to make my nipples bleed, a feat I never knew was possible. (Breastfeeding moms are yelling at me from the street. Also, nice job multitasking, reading this book and breastfeeding, moms!)

And frankly, people find me more attractive now than when I was someone who didn't care at all about his diet or exercise. Whether it's because of actually changing how my body looks or the confidence I've gained by pushing myself and caring more about how I look, it's been helpful in social situations, as well as in my dating life. (Hello to any current and future love interests!)

On top of that, I've proved to myself that if I want to lose weight, or if I want to become more athletic, or if I have any sort of fitness goal, I can accomplish it. I've done it many times over the course of the year and a half I spent writing this book. I've also seen others accomplish their goals, at all different ages, and that's helped push me and remind me that anything is possible. That will never leave my brain. (Hopefully.)

I also learned what types of exercise I like. Who knew that I would actually enjoy running a lot? Who knew that rock climbing would be scary and fun, or a spin class would be pure torture? Or that I would grow to love the camaraderie of group fitness classes and CrossFit? Or that there's more to life than just lifting weights at a gym while blasting loud music in my headphones?

I also learned what not to do—don't jump from thing to thing. While researching this book, I would be into half-marathon training for a period of time. Then I'd be into lifting heavy weights. Then I'd do CrossFit. Or yoga. Or something else.

Because I hopped from program to program, from goal to goal, my results weren't always as consistent. I got the best results when I focused on one thing instead of trying to do ALL THE THINGS.

Perhaps most important, I learned that the person I used to

be—the obese, most likely pre-diabetic man who couldn't find pants anywhere—wasn't a failure. I wasn't some morally repugnant blight on society because of my weight—and neither is anyone else.

The modern food system is geared toward making you fat. Our jobs and where we live are geared toward making us fat. *Most exercise-oriented businesses don't actually help make you less fat.*

On top of that, *your body wants you to be fatter.* The whole system is rigged against us. And then we act as if it's *our* fault, *our* failure, when all these other factors come into play.

Life isn't fair. But we can at least stop judging one another over stupid shit like our bodies.

Plus I learned that your health and well-being are not defined by a number on a scale. People can be obese but still be much healthier than folks who are considered skinny. You can be healthy at a lot of different sizes.

And regardless of your weight, or your body-fat percentage, or how much you can deadlift, you're deserving of love.

Here are a few things I hope you learned from this book:

1. Some new skills to set you up for success for your fitness goals.
2. That losing weight isn't the be-all, end-all for fitness.
3. Fitness is a lifelong journey, and you may change your mind about what your goals are.
4. Motivation comes from within, but external factors are also important.
5. No matter where you start, you are capable of doing great things with your body, and if you stumble during your journey, that's not only okay, but it's normal.
6. If you are overweight or unhealthy, it's not all your fault. You

live in a society that wants you to be overweight. Skinny people are the aberration. You can be healthy and still be "fat."

7. Above all else, love yourself.

I set out to write a book about fitness and weight loss from the vantage point of someone who spent the majority of his life as a fat guy. If you walk through the fitness section of most book stores, you see all these hunky men and gorgeous women staring back at you on book covers, a bunch of ripped humans with washboard abs, shoulders popping like daggers, and curves that could take out a bus, and they act as if they know the same struggles as those of us who've spent our lives a little less physically fit. I wanted to write a book that would resonate with the majority of people who are like me.

I also wanted to spend a year making my body look better and losing some weight. How did I do in that goal? Well, the most I lost was twenty-five pounds after my second half marathon. I'm currently, as I write this, hovering at about twenty pounds below my starting weight.

Maybe more than anything, I changed how I viewed my body. It's no longer as important for me to look fantastic in a T-shirt. Sure, it's a nice goal, and a lot of the things I've done in the past year have helped me look better, in some respects.

But you know what's cooler? Being strong. Running long distances. Getting better at things. Having the ability to do activities I never thought I could do. It's now more about functionality than it is about vanity. A bonus is that in the event of a total societal collapse, I'm now more likely to survive the nightmarish hellscape.

I'm happy about that. (I mean, not the potential for a dystopian future, but everything else.) I hope you come to find something similar in your fitness goals—as you work toward having a better-functioning body, however you want to define that.

Maybe it's so you can shoot hoops with friends and be less out of breath. Maybe it's so you can chase after your kids at the end of a long workday. Maybe it's so you can feel more confident in your body.

Whatever your goals, make it about something you can test, or a goal you make within yourself. You can't control how people view your body, even after all the hard work you put in. But you *can* work toward becoming stronger, faster, or more flexible.

I hope you've learned—and laughed—from my mistakes. I hope you've discovered that getting on a better path toward fitness just requires that you take a few small steps at a time, that it's a journey you'll spend the rest of your life doing, and that when combined, those small steps turn into miles and miles and miles. (Or kilometers, for anyone who isn't American.)

I hope you learned that it is worth it to spend some extra time taking care of yourself. That you are worthy of love, no matter how you look, no matter your level of physical ability, no matter anything.

But overall, I hope you have learned to believe in yourself. Because I believe in you.

—Andy Boyle

Acknowledgments

No one succeeds in a vacuum, and I am a testament to that. This book wouldn't have been possible without the help of many wonderfully talented people.

Thanks go to my agent, Noah Ballard, for believing in the project. My editors, Lauren Appleton and Marian Lizzi, for pushing me to make the best book possible. M.P. Klier for her amazing copy editing and saving my butt more than once. Everyone else at Penguin Random House and TarcherPerigee who helped promote and make this book a reality. Thank you for giving me not one but *two* chances at putting my thoughts and ideas into the universe in book form.

Thanks to all my friends who read early drafts and offered notes: Emily "Grafflebagel" Greenhalgh, Bryan Duffy, Stephanie Kubik, Felipe Cabrera, and S. Baer Lederman. And thanks to Teagan Walsh-Davis, who also read it and was a tremendous help. You're the best ex-girlfriend a guy could have.

Thanks to my family for dealing with my needing to eat healthy or go to the gym during "family vacation time." Thanks to my coworkers, as well as my former bosses (shout-outs to Matt Boggie and Josh Sloat) for not getting mad if I went to the gym during my lunch break or went for a training run when work got slow.

Thank you to the various medical professionals who took time to talk with me or just treat me in general over the years, including Dr. Dan Jacobazzi, who owned the first gym I ever felt comfortable in.

And to the guy who told me in college I'd never run a half marathon because I was too fat: Not only did I run two, but I got *paid* to run them. Thanks for the motivation.

Final thanks go to you, too, dear reader. Supporting books is awesome, and by getting this far, it usually means you read the dang thing. Hopefully you learned a thing or two and it was helpful, even just a little bit. If you liked the book, tell all your friends. If you didn't, that's okay! Tell people to read something else then. Just keep reading.

Notes

2. How America—and the World—Got Fat

1. Anne Hollander, "When Fat Was in Fashion," *New York Times,* October 23, 1977, accessed June 2, 2019, https://www.nytimes.com/1977/10/23/archives/when -fat-was-in-fashion-abundant-flesh-was-a-thing-of-beauty-to.html.
2. "The History of Obesity—the Renaissance to 1910," SERMO, June 22, 2015, accessed June 2, 2019, http://blog.sermo.com/2015/07/02/history-obesity -renaissance-1910/.
3. Garabed Eknoyan, "A History of Obesity, or How What Was Good Became Ugly and Then Bad," *Advances in Chronic Kidney Disease* 13, no. 4 (October 2006): 421–27, accessed June 2, 2019, doi:10.1053/j.ackd.2006.07.002.
4. Natalie Wolchover, "The Real Skinny: Expert Traces America's Thin Obsession," LiveScience, January 26, 2012, accessed June 2, 2019, https://www .livescience.com/18131-women-thin-dieting-history.html.
5. Dean Baker and Nick Buffie, "The Decline of Blue-Collar Jobs, in Graphs," Center for Economic and Policy Research Blog, February 22, 2017, accessed June 2, 2019, http://cepr.net/blogs/cepr-blog/the-decline-of-blue-collar-jobs-in-graphs.
6. "Farm Labor," United States Department of Agriculture Economic Research Service, accessed June 2, 2019, https://www.ers.usda.gov/topics/farm -economy/farm-labor/#size.
7. Marc Cenedella, "Great News! We've Become a White-Collar Nation," *Business Insider,* January 7, 2010, accessed June 2, 2019, https://www.businessinsider .com/great-news-weve-become-a-white-collar-nation-2010-1.
8. "How Color Affects Your Appetite," Care2 Healthy Living, November 6, 2015, accessed June 2, 2019, https://www.care2.com/greenliving/how-color-affects -your-appetite.html.
9. Eric H. Chudler, "Does the Color of Foods and Drinks Affect the Sense of Taste?" Neuroscience for Kids, accessed June 2, 2019, https://faculty .washington.edu/chudler/coltaste.html.
10. Ittersum, Koert Van, and Brian Wansink. "Plate Size and Color Suggestibility: The Delboeuf Illusion's Bias on Serving and Eating Behavior." *Journal of Consumer Research* 39, no. 2 (August 1, 2012): 215–28. https://doi.org/10.1086 /662615.

11. Benjamin F. Evans, Emily Zimmerman, Steven H. Woolf, and Amber D. Haley, *Food Access and Health in Cook County, Illinois,* Virginia Commonwealth University Center on Human Needs, July 2012, accessed June 2, 2019, https://societyhealth.vcu.edu/media/society-health/pdf/PMReport_Cook_Co.pdf.
12. Pianin, Eric. "Billions in Tax Dollars Subsidize Junk Food Industry." The Fiscal Times. July 25, 2012. Accessed August 22, 2019. https://www.thefiscaltimes.com/Articles/2012/07/25/Billions-in-Tax-Dollars-Subsidize-Junk-Food-Industry.
13. James A. Levine, "Poverty and Obesity in the U.S," figure 1, *Diabetes* 60, no. 11 (2011): 2667–68, accessed June 2, 2019, doi:10.2337/db11-1118.

3. Marketing Your Health, or Big Wellness Takes Over

1. Jennie Dusheck and Christopher Silas Neal, "The Science of Wellness," *Stanford Medicine,* 2016, accessed June 2, 2019, https://stanmed.stanford.edu/2016summer/well-now.html.
2. Stef W. Kight, "Fitness Industry Booms, but We're Not Getting Fitter," Axios, October 22, 2018, accessed June 2, 2019, https://www.axios.com/health-wellness-obesity-fat-weight-gain-loss-diet-industry-8b1f4fa4-0299-4986-9544-61af14786b1a.html.
3. Yvette D'Entremont, "The Sickening Business of Wellness," *The Outline,* December 13, 2016, accessed June 2, 2019, https://theoutline.com/post/350/the-sickening-business-of-wellness?zd=1&zi=qku5bj7l.
4. Laura Clark, "How Halitosis Became a Medical Condition with a 'Cure,'" Smithsonian.com, January 29, 2015, accessed June 2, 2019, https://www.smithsonianmag.com/smart-news/marketing-campaign-invented-halitosis-180954082/.
5. "U.S. Weight Loss Market Worth $66 Billion," PR Newswire, June 26, 2018, accessed June 2, 2019, https://www.prnewswire.com/news-releases/us-weight-loss-market-worth-66-billion-300573968.html.
6. Lisa Hix, "How Snake Oil Got a Bad Rap (Hint: It Wasn't the Snakes' Fault)," Collectors Weekly, March 20, 2011, accessed June 2, 2019, https://www.collectorsweekly.com/articles/how-snake-oil-got-a-bad-rap/.
7. Max Rothman, "Red Bull to Pay $13 Million for False Advertising Settlement," BevNET.com, September 10, 2015, accessed June 2, 2019, https://www.bevnet.com/news/2014/red-bull-to-pay-13-million-for-false-advertising-settlement.
8. Missy Schwartz, "Got Milk? How the Iconic Campaign Came to Be, 25 Years Ago," *Fast Company,* July 6, 2018, accessed June 2, 2019, https://www.fastcompany.com/40556502/got-milk-how-the-iconic-campaign-came-to-be-25-years-ago.
9. Mary L. Garcia-Cazarin, Edwina A. Wambogo, Karen S. Regan, and Cindy D. Davis, "Dietary Supplement Research Portfolio at the NIH, 2009–2011," *Journal of Nutrition* 144, no. 4 (April 2014): 414–18, doi:10.3945/jn.113.189803.
10. Lawson, K. A., M. E. Wright, A. Subar, T. Mouw, A. Hollenbeck, A. Schatzkin, and M. F. Leitzmann. "Multivitamin Use and Risk of Prostate Cancer in the National Institutes of Health-AARP Diet and Health Study." *JNCI Journal of the National Cancer Institute* 99, no. 10 (May 15, 2007): 754–64. https://doi.org/10.1093/jnci/djk177.

11. "A.G. Schneiderman Asks Major Retailers To Halt Sales Of Certain." New York State Attorney General. February 3, 2015. Accessed June 02, 2019. https://ag.ny .gov/press-release/ag-schneiderman-asks-major-retailers-halt-sales-certain -herbal-supplements-dna-tests.

12. Daniel Duane, "Everything You Know About Fitness Is a Lie," *Men's Journal*, December 4, 2017, accessed June 2, 2019, https://www.mensjournal.com /features/everything-you-know-about-fitness-is-a-lie-20120504/.

13. Harry Bradford, "Abercrombie & Fitch's Reputation Takes A Hit After CEO's 'Fat' Comments Resurface," *Huffington Post*, December 7, 2017, accessed June 2, 2019, https://www.huffingtonpost.com/2013/05/16/abercrombie-reputation -ceo-comments_n_3288836.html.

14. Nadra Nittle, "Women's Clothing Is Divided into Straight and Plus Sizes. Here's Why That's a Problem," *Vox*, October 12, 2018, accessed June 2, 2019, https:// www.vox.com/the-goods/2018/10/12/17969968/womens-clothing-sizes -divided-straight-sizes-plus-sizes-universal-standard-clothing-segregation.

15. "New Statistics Reveal the Shape of Plastic Surgery," American Society of Plastic Surgeons, March 1, 2018, accessed June 2, 2019, https://www .plasticsurgery.org/news/press-releases/new-statistics-reveal-the-shape-of -plastic-surgery.

16. Mayo Clinic Staff, "Liposuction," Mayo Clinic, February 26, 2019, accessed June 2, 2019, https://www.mayoclinic.org/tests-procedures/liposuction/about /pac-20384586.

4. What Is Actually *in* Food, Anyway?

1. Drew DeSilver, "How America's Diet Has Changed Over Time," Pew Research Center, December 13, 2016, accessed June 2, 2019, https://www.pewresearch .org/fact-tank/2016/12/13/whats-on-your-table-how-americas-diet-has -changed-over-the-decades/.

2. Eurídice Martínez Steele, Larissa Galastri Baraldi, Maria Laura Da Costa Lou-zada, Jean-Claude Moubarac, Dariush Mozaffarian, and Carlos Augusto Monteiro, "Ultra-processed Foods and Added Sugars in the US Diet: Evidence from a Nationally Representative Cross-Sectional Study," *BMJ Open* 6, no. 3 (2016), accessed June 2, 2019, doi:10.1136/bmjopen-2015-009892.

3. Saksena, Michelle J., Abigail M. Okrent, Tobenna D. Anekwe, and Et Al. "America's Eating Habits: Food Away From Home." United States Department of Agriculture Economic Research Service, September 2018. September 2018. Accessed June 2, 2019. https://www.ers.usda.gov/webdocs/publications/90228 /eib-196_summary.pdf?v=1045.6.

4. Julia A. Wolfson and Sara N. Bleich, "Is Cooking at Home Associated with Better Diet Quality or Weight-Loss Intention?," *Public Health Nutrition* 18, no. 8 (2014): 1397–406, June 2015, accessed June 2, 2019, doi:10.1017 /s1368980014001943.

5. Kim Parker, "Women Still Bear Heavier Load Than Men in Balancing Work, Family," Pew Research Center, March 10, 2015, accessed June 2, 2019, https:// www.pewresearch.org/fact-tank/2015/03/10/women-still-bear-heavier-load -than-men-balancing-work-family/.

6. DeSilver, "How America's Diet Has Changed Over Time."

7. Erica M. Schulte, Nicole M. Avena, and Ashley N. Gearhardt, "Which Foods May Be Addictive? The Roles of Processing, Fat Content, and Glycemic Load," *PLOS One* 10, no. 2 (February 18, 2015), accessed June 2, 2019, doi:10.1371/journal.pone.0117959.

8. George Dvorsky, "How Flavor Chemists Make Your Food So Addictively Good," *Io9*, December 16, 2015, accessed June 2, 2019, https://io9.gizmodo.com/5958880/how-flavor-chemists-make-your-food-so-addictively-good.

9. Nancy Luna, "Doritos Taco Most Successful Taco Bell Product—Ever," *Orange County Register*, June 4, 2012, accessed June 2, 2019, https://www.ocregister.com/2012/06/04/doritos-taco-most-successful-taco-bell-product-ever/.

10. "Taco Bell's Newest Menu Item Now Its Highest Selling," *New York Post*, March 14, 2018, accessed June 2, 2019, https://nypost.com/2018/03/14/taco-bells-newest-menu-item-now-its-highest-selling/.

11. Kelly Tyko, "Burger King Says Its New Halloween Creation 'Nightmare King' Can Induce Nightmares," *USA Today*, October 27, 2018, accessed June 2, 2019, https://www.usatoday.com/story/money/2018/10/17/burger-king-nightmare-king-halloween/1661125002/.

12. Richard D. Mattes, Penny M. Kris-Etherton, and Gary D. Foster, "Impact of Peanuts and Tree Nuts on Body Weight and Healthy Weight Loss in Adults," *Journal of Nutrition*, September 1, 2008, accessed June 2, 2019, https://www.ncbi.nlm.nih.gov/pubmed/18716179.

13. Baer, David J., Sarah K. Gebauer, and Janet A. Novotny. "Measured Energy Value of Pistachios in the Human Diet." *British Journal of Nutrition* 107, no. 1 (June 28, 2011): 120–25. https://doi.org/10.1017/s0007114511002649.

14. Madison Park, "Twinkie Diet Helps Nutrition Professor Lose 27 Pounds," CNN, November 8, 2010, accessed June 2, 2019, http://www.cnn.com/2010/HEALTH/11/08/twinkie.diet.professor/index.html.

15. "Alcohol Facts and Statistics," National Institute on Alcohol Abuse and Alcoholism, August 2018, accessed June 2, 2019, https://www.niaaa.nih.gov/alcohol-health/overview-alcohol-consumption/alcohol-facts-and-statistics.

5. Your Body, Explained

1. Church, Timothy S., Conrad P. Earnest, James S. Skinner, and Steven N. Blair. "Effects of Different Doses of Physical Activity on Cardiorespiratory Fitness Among Sedentary, Overweight or Obese Postmenopausal Women With Elevated Blood Pressure." *JAMA* 297, no. 19 (May 16, 2007): 2081. https://doi.org/10.1001/jama.297.19.2081.

2. Druce, M. R., A. M. Wren, A. J. Park, J. E. Milton, M. Patterson, G. Frost, M. A. Ghatei, C. Small, and S. R. Bloom. "Ghrelin Increases Food Intake in Obese as Well as Lean Subjects." *International Journal of Obesity* 29, no. 9 (September 2005): 1130-136. Accessed June 2, 2019. doi:10.1038/sj.ijo.0803001.

3. Cynthia Ogden and Margaret Carroll, "Prevalence of Obesity Among Children and Adolescents: United States, Trends 1963–1965 Through 2007–2008," PsycEXTRA Dataset, September 2014, accessed June 2, 2019, doi:10.1037/e582042012-001.

4. Roland Sturm and Ruopeng An, "Obesity and Economic Environments," *CA: A*

Cancer Journal for Clinicians 64, no. 5 (September 2014): 337–50, accessed June 2, 2019, doi:10.3322/caac.21237.

5. "Direct-to-Consumer Genetic Tests." Consumer Information. Federal Trade Commission, March 13, 2018. https://www.consumer.ftc.gov/articles/0166 -direct-consumer-genetic-tests.

6. Chris Welch, "FDA Orders 23andMe to Halt Sales of DNA Test Kit," The Verge, November 25, 2013, accessed June 3, 2019, https://www.theverge.com/2013/11 /25/5143464/fda-orders-23andme-to-stop-selling-dna-test-kit.

7. Heather Murphy, "How an Unlikely Family History Website Transformed Cold Case Investigations," *New York Times*, October 15, 2018, accessed June 2, 2019, https://www.nytimes.com/2018/10/15/science/gedmatch-genealogy-cold-cases .html.

8. Peter Aldhous, "This Genealogy Database Helped Solve Dozens of Crimes. But Its New Privacy Rules Will Restrict Access by Cops," BuzzFeed News, May 21, 2019, accessed June 3, 2019, https://www.buzzfeednews.com/article /peteraldhous/this-genealogy-database-helped-solve-dozens-of-crimes-but.

9. American Thoracic Society, "Sleeping Less Linked to Weight Gain," Science-Daily, May 29, 2006, accessed June 2, 2019, www.sciencedaily.com/releases /2006/05/060529082903.htm.

10. Marek Ruchała, Barbara Bromińska, Ewa Cyrańska-Chyrek, Barbara Kuźnar-Kamińska, Magdalena Kostrzewska, and Halina Batura-Gabryel, "Obstructive Sleep Apnea and Hormones—a Novel Insight," *Archives of Medical Science* 4 (June 2017): 875–84, accessed June 2, 2019, doi:10.5114/aoms.2016.61499.

11. Thomas G. Travison, Andre B. Araujo, Amy B. O'Donnell, Varant Kupelian, and John B. McKinlay, "A Population-Level Decline in Serum Testosterone Levels in American Men," *Journal of Clinical Endocrinology and Metabolism* 92, no. 1 (January 2007): 196–202, accessed June 2, 2019, doi:10.1210/jc.2006-1375.

12. Erlingur Nordal, "Testosterone Levels Decreasing in Danish Men," IceNews, May 17, 2010, accessed June 2, 2019, https://www.icenews.is/2010/05/17 /testosterone-levels-decreasing-in-danish-men/#axzz4f1HF2xrr.

6. How to Know if Someone Is Vegan (and Other Diets, Explained)

1. Charlotte Edwardes, "Mr Banting's Old Diet Revolution," *Telegraph*, September 14, 2003, accessed June 2, 2019, https://www.telegraph.co.uk/news /uknews/1441407/Mr-Bantings-Old-Diet-Revolution.html.

2. Joy Wilke, "Nearly Half in U.S. Remain Worried About Their Weight," Gallup .com, July 25, 2014, accessed June 2, 2019, https://news.gallup.com/poll/174089 /nearly-half-remain-worried-weight.aspx.

3. Fildes, Alison, Judith Charlton, Caroline Rudisill, Peter Littlejohns, A Toby Prevost, and Martin C Gulliford. "Probability of an Obese Person Attaining Normal Body Weight: Cohort Study Using Electronic Health Records." *American Journal of Public Health*. American Public Health Association, September 2015. https://www.ncbi.nlm.nih.gov/pmc/articles/PMC4539812/.

4. Collier, R. "Intermittent Fasting: The Science of Going without." *Canadian Medical Association Journal* 185, no. 9 (June 11, 2013). Accessed August 21, 2019. doi:10.1503/cmaj.109-4451.

5. Christian Zauner, Bruno Schneeweiss, Alexander Kranz, Christian Madl, Klaus Ratheiser, Ludwig Kramer, Erich Roth, Barbara Schneider, and Kurt Lenz, "Resting Energy Expenditure in Short-Term Starvation Is Increased as a Result of an Increase in Serum Norepinephrine," *American Journal of Clinical Nutrition* 71, no. 6 (June 2000): 1511–15, accessed June 2, 2019, doi:10.1093/ajcn/71.6.1511.

6. Barnosky, Adrienne R., Kristin K. Hoddy, Terry G. Unterman, and Krista A. Varady. "Intermittent Fasting vs Daily Calorie Restriction for Type 2 Diabetes Prevention: A Review of Human Findings." *Translational Research* 164, no. 4 (October 2014): 302-11. Accessed August 21, 2019. doi:10.1016/j.trsl.2014.05.013.

7. Li, Liaoliao, Zhi Wang, and Zhiyi Zuo. "Chronic Intermittent Fasting Improves Cognitive Functions and Brain Structures in Mice." *PLoS ONE* 8, no. 6 (June 03, 2013). Accessed August 21, 2019. doi:10.1371/journal.pone.0066069.

8. Faris, "Moez Al-Islam" E., Safia Kacimi, Refat A. Al-Kurd, Mohammad A. Fararjeh, Yasser K. Bustanji, Mohammad K. Mohammad, and Mohammad L. Salem. "Intermittent Fasting during Ramadan Attenuates Proinflammatory Cytokines and Immune Cells in Healthy Subjects." *Nutrition Research* 32, no. 12 (December 2012): 947-55. Accessed August 21, 2019. doi:10.1016/j.nutres.2012.06.021.

9. Horne, Benjamin D., Heidi T. May, Jeffrey L. Anderson, Abdallah G. Kfoury, Beau M. Bailey, Brian S. Mcclure, Dale G. Renlund, Donald L. Lappé, John F. Carlquist, Patrick W. Fisher, Robert R. Pearson, Tami L. Bair, Ted D. Adams, and Joseph B. Muhlestein. "Usefulness of Routine Periodic Fasting to Lower Risk of Coronary Artery Disease in Patients Undergoing Coronary Angiography." *The American Journal of Cardiology* 102, no. 7 (October 2008). Accessed August 21, 2019. doi:10.1016/j.amjcard.2008.05.021.

10. Goodrick, Charles L., Donald K. Ingram, Mark A. Reynolds, John R. Freeman, and Nancy L. Cider. "Effects of Intermittent Feeding Upon Growth and Life Span in Rats." *Gerontology* 28, no. 4 (1982): 233-41. Accessed August 21, 2019. doi:10.1159/000212538.

11. Marcelo Campos, "Ketogenic Diet: Is the Ultimate Low-Carb Diet Good for You?," Harvard Health Blog, July 6, 2018, accessed June 2, 2019, https://www.health.harvard.edu/blog/ketogenic-diet-is-the-ultimate-low-carb-diet-good-for-you-2017072712089.

12. Dashti, Hussein M., Naji S. Al-Zaid, Thazhumpal C. Mathew, Mahdi Al-Mousawi, Hussain Talib, Sami K. Asfar, and Abdulla I. Behbahani. "Long Term Effects of Ketogenic Diet in Obese Subjects with High Cholesterol Level." *Molecular and Cellular Biochemistry* 286, no. 1-2 (June 21, 2006): 1-9. Accessed August 21, 2019. doi:10.1007/s11010-005-9001-x.

7. Exercise Is Important, but How Important, Really?

1. Timothy S. Church, Conrad P. Earnest, James S. Skinner, and Steven N. Blair, "Effects of Different Doses of Physical Activity on Cardiorespiratory Fitness Among Sedentary, Overweight or Obese Postmenopausal Women with Elevated Blood Pressure," *JAMA* 297, no. 19 (May 2007): 2081, accessed June 2, 2019, doi:10.1001/jama.297.19,2081.

2. Amy Marturana, "How Alison Brie Got in Fighting Shape for 'GLOW,'" *Self*, July 10, 2017, accessed June 2, 2019, https://www.self.com/story/alison-brie-glow-workout.

3. Stephanie Chan, "How Alison Brie Got in Fighting Shape for Netflix's 'Glow,'" *Hollywood Reporter*, May 25, 2017, accessed June 2, 2019, https://www.hollywoodreporter.com/news/netflix-glow-alison-brie-training-role-1007308.

4. "Our Studios," SoulCycle, accessed June 2, 2019, https://www.soul-cycle.com/studios/all/.

5. Patrick J. O'Connor, Matthew P. Herring, and Amanda Caravalho, "Mental Health Benefits of Strength Training in Adults," *American Journal of Lifestyle Medicine* 4, no. 5 (2010): 377–96, accessed June 2, 2019, doi:10.1177/1559827610368771.

6. Brett R. Gordon, Cillian P. McDowell, Mats Hallgren, Jacob D. Meyer, Mark Lyons, and Matthew P. Herring, "Association of Efficacy of Resistance Exercise Training with Depressive Symptoms," *JAMA Psychiatry* 75, no. 6 (June 1, 2018): 566, accessed June 2, 2019, doi:10.1001/jamapsychiatry.2018.0572.

8. Mental Health and How It Impacts Your Weight (and Beyond!)

1. "Facts and Statistics," Anxiety and Depression Association of America, accessed June 2, 2019, https://adaa.org/about-adaa/press-room/facts-statistics.

2. "Depression," Anxiety and Depression Association of America, accessed June 2, 2019, https://adaa.org/understanding-anxiety/depression.

3. "UN Health Agency Reports Depression Now 'Leading Cause of Disability Worldwide' | UN News." United Nations. February 23, 2017. Accessed August 21, 2019. https://news.un.org/en/story/2017/02/552062-un-health-agency-reports-depression-now-leading-cause-disability-worldwide#.WLRpQBB3xBw.

4. David Engstrom, "Obesity and Depression," Obesity Action Coalition, accessed June 2, 2019, https://www.obesityaction.org/community/article-library/obesity-and-depression/.

5. S. Virk, T. L. Schwartz, S. Jindal, N. Nihalani, and N. Jones, "Psychiatric Medication Induced Obesity: An Aetiologic Review," *Obesity Reviews* 5, no. 3 (May 2004): 167–70, accessed June 2, 2019, doi:10.1111/j.1467-789x.2004.00141.x.

6. Jun Yan, "Percentage of Americans Taking Antidepressants Climbs," *Psychiatric News*, September 15, 2017, accessed June 2, 2019, https://psychnews.psychiatryonline.org/doi/full/10.1176/appi.pn.2017.pp9b2.

7. Thomas J. Moore and Donald R. Mattison, "Adult Utilization of Psychiatric Drugs and Differences by Sex, Age, and Race," *JAMA Internal Medicine* 177, no. 2 (February 2017): 274, accessed June 2, 2019, doi:10.1001/jamainternmed.2016.7507.

8. Emily Nagoski, "The Science of (Sexual) Frustration," *Dirty Normal*, May 25, 2014, accessed June 2, 2019, https://thedirtynormal.com/post/2014/05/28/the-science-of-sexual-frustration.

9. Alberga, Angela S., Shelly Russell-Mayhew, Kristin M. Von Ranson, and Lindsay McLaren. "Weight Bias: A Call to Action." *Journal of Eating Disorders*. November 07, 2016. Accessed August 21, 2019. https://www.ncbi.nlm.nih.gov/pmc/articles/PMC5100338/.

10. Angela S. Alberga, Shelly Russell-Mayhew, Kristin M. Von Ranson, and Lindsay McLaren, "Weight Bias: A Call to Action," *Journal of Eating Disorders* 4, no. 1 (November 7, 2016), accessed June 2, 2019, doi:10.1186/s40337-016-0112-4.

11. Rheana Murray, "Where's the Least Body-Positive State in America? You Might Be Surprised," Today.com, May 8, 2018, accessed June 2, 2019, https://www.today.com/style/social-media-affecting-way-we-view-our-bodies-it-s-t128500.

12. Mark D. Griffiths, "Addicted to Social Media?" *Psychology Today*, May 7, 2018, accessed June 2, 2019, https://www.psychologytoday.com/us/blog/in-excess/201805/addicted-social-media.

13. Editors, "What We Learned About Sexual Desire from 10 Years of Pornhub User Data," *The Cut*, June 11, 2017, accessed June 2, 2019, https://www.thecut.com/2017/06/pornhub-data-sexual-habits.html.

14. Katherine Sellgren, "Pornography 'Desensitising Young People,'" BBC News, June 15, 2016, accessed June 2, 2019, https://www.bbc.com/news/education-36527681.

15. Diller, Vivian. "Internet Porn and Body Image." *Psychology Today*. September 4, 2012. Accessed June 2, 2019. https://www.psychologytoday.com/us/blog/face-it/201209/internet-porn-and-body-image.

9. The How-To Part of the Book

1. Elisabet Børsheim and Roald Bahr, "Effect of Exercise Intensity, Duration and Mode on Post-Exercise Oxygen Consumption," *Sports Medicine* 33, no. 14 (2003): 1037–60, accessed June 2, 2019, doi:10.2165/00007256-200333140-00002.

2. Stephan Von Haehling, John E. Morley, and Stefan D. Anker, "An Overview of Sarcopenia: Facts and Numbers on Prevalence and Clinical Impact," *Journal of Cachexia, Sarcopenia and Muscle* 1, no. 2 (December 2010): 129–33, doi:10.1007/s13539-010-0014-2.

3. "Physical Activity Guidelines for Americans," HHS.gov, February 1, 2019, accessed June 2, 2019, https://www.hhs.gov/fitness/be-active/physical-activity-guidelines-for-americans/index.html.

4. Derek Thompson, "The Myth That Americans Are Busier Than Ever," *Atlantic*, May 21, 2014, accessed June 2, 2019, https://www.theatlantic.com/business/archive/2014/05/the-myth-that-americans-are-busier-than-ever/371350/.

About the Author

Andy Boyle is an award-winning journalist and web developer. He is also the author of *Adulthood for Beginners: All the Life Secrets Nobody Bothered to Tell You*. He's previously worked with the *Chicago Sun-Times*, Axios, NBC News, the *Chicago Tribune*, the *Boston Globe*, the *Tampa Bay Times,* and The New York Times Regional Media Group, where a project of his was cited in the 2012 Pulitzer Prize for Breaking News Reporting. He lives in Chicago, where he likes running outside, even in the winter.